# A Practical Guide to Clinical Ethics Consulting

# A Practical Guide to Clinical Ethics Consulting

*Expertise, Ethos, and Power*

Christopher Meyers

ROWMAN & LITTLEFIELD PUBLISHERS, INC.
Lanham • Boulder • New York • Toronto • Plymouth, UK

ROWMAN & LITTLEFIELD PUBLISHERS, INC.

Published in the United States of America
by Rowman & Littlefield Publishers, Inc.
A wholly owned subsidiary of The Rowman & Littlefield Publishing Group, Inc.
4501 Forbes Boulevard, Suite 200, Lanham, Maryland 20706
www.rowmanlittlefield.com

Estover Road
Plymouth PL6 7PY
United Kingdom

British Library Cataloguing in Publication Information Available

**Library of Congress Cataloging-in-Publication Data:**
Meyers, Christopher, 1957–
   A practical guide to clinical ethics consulting : expertise, ethos, and power /
Christopher Meyers.
      p. ; cm.
   Includes index.
   ISBN-13: 978-0-7425-4827-5 (cloth : alk. paper)
   ISBN-10: 0-7425-4827-9 (cloth : alk. paper)
   ISBN-13: 978-0-7425-4828-2 (pbk. : alk. paper)
   ISBN-10: 0-7425-4828-7 (pbk. : alk. paper)
   1. Medical ethics. 2. Medical ethics—Social aspects. I. Title.
   [DNLM: 1. Ethics, Clinical. 2. Ethical Review. WB 60 M613p 2007]

R724.M438 2007
174.2—dc22                                          2007005736

Printed in the United States of America

⊗™ The paper used in this publication meets the minimum requirements of
American National Standard for Information Sciences—Permanence of Paper
for Printed Library Materials, ANSI/NISO Z39.48-1992.

For Renee, Jon, and Natasha, and
especially for Donna,
for creating the joyful life
through which good work can emerge.

# Contents

# Acknowledgments

Most of the critical work for this book was completed during visiting scholar appointments at the Centre for Applied Philosophy and Public Ethics and at The Hastings Center. I am deeply grateful to both centers for providing dedicated research and writing time and to the resident scholars for their always helpful criticism and great companionship. Individual acknowledgments are noted throughout the book, but special thanks are owed to Seumas Miller, Keith Horton, and Peter Roberts, from CAPPE; and to Dan Callahan, Bette-Jane Crigger, and Bruce Jennings, at Hastings.

I am also indebted to David Adams, Glenn Graber, and Lisa Parker for their insightful reviews; the book is much better for their recommendations.

The earliest seeds of the book are rooted in my struggle with how to be a sympathetic, even empathetic, clinical advisor while also retaining critical independence. The many physicians, nurses, and hospital administrators with whom I have worked over the years regularly reinforce the need for such empathy, given their caring commitment to patients' well-being. At the same time, my philosophy colleagues have steadily reinforced the need for independence. Both motivations have been critical to how I think about and practice clinical ethics. I thank you all.

~

# Introduction

Consider the following list: "the herbologist and the golf pro, the pollster and the journalism professor, the Feng Shui counselor and the aroma therapist, . . . and the bioethicist." What do its items have in common? According to Andrew Ferguson, they are all occupations whose practitioners' labor "would be regarded as frivolous at best, freeloading at worst . . . in a country less indulgent, less able to tolerate excess baggage, less rolling in the dough." Such practitioners are, in short, "spongers," about whom "you can't help but wonder, [what] are they good for?"[1]

These comments come from the opening of Ferguson's review of Leon Kass's *Life, Liberty, and the Defense of Dignity*,[2] and they capture Kass's critical tone toward current practice in bioethics, especially toward the idea that academic (read: philosophical) training makes one an ethics expert.[3] Rather, Kass argues, academic training produces mainly *meta*-ethicists, people who seek

> to analyze and clarify moral argumentation; to establish or criticize grounds for justifying our decisions; to lay down rules and guidelines, principles and procedures, for addressing ethical dilemmas; and, in some cases, to construct comprehensive theories of conduct centering around fundamental norms, called "autonomy" or "utility" or "duty" or "equality" or "beneficence."[4]

Academic training, in other words, produces people skilled at *talking about* doing ethics, rather than skilled at actually doing it. Philosophers, so Kass suggests, are too abstract, too hung up on conceptual niceties to get at what is at stake in real ethical problems.

1

Variants on this criticism have been present in the literature for years and are exemplified in Barry Hoffmaster's oft-quoted "Can Ethnography Save the Life of Medical Ethics?": "The principles standardly regarded as constituting the core of theoretical medical ethics . . . are too general and vague to apply determinately to concrete situations. . . . The real culprit . . . is a philosophical approach that creates and sustains the impression that moral theory and moral practice are discrete."[5] Moral theorists (on the whole philosophers) cannot, the argument goes, hope to provide useful, action-guiding models through a priori reasoning. Rather, moral reasoning must be explicitly and directly informed by the *real*, by the day-to-day tangible struggles of practitioners. While practice without theory is strictly ad hoc, theory without practice is merely abstract, devoid of the reality necessary to guide human choices.

Furthermore, the critique continues, even when they get it right intellectually, there is no assurance philosophers will be able to act on such knowledge in the appropriate ways. That is, despite Socrates' claims to the contrary, there is no essential connection between moral knowledge and moral virtue. Philosophers are just as likely to be morally corrupt, indeed maybe even more so. If anything, the more predominant fear is the one regularly, and only half-jokingly, expressed by introductory ethics students—that being proficient at ethical analysis makes one more skilled at rationalizing one's behavior. And even when knowledgeable and virtuous, philosophers may well lack other skills critical to clinical ethics, for example, effective communication, including the ability to translate complex abstractions into ordinary, accessible language, and political sophistication, so as to manage the politics of rigidly hierarchical institutions like hospitals.

It is not surprising, then, that the last decade has seen many business and professional organizations rejecting philosopher-ethicists as consultants, preferring instead to send an in-house person to one- or two-week ethics education programs. Doing this, they believe, gives them a person trained in ethics and grounded in the organization's specific practice.

In short, the attacks on philosophers as clinical ethicists are many and come from multiple quarters. Are they right? My argument in this book is they are, but only partly so and not in the most important respects. They are right in that practical ethics that relies too heavily on conceptual analysis is of little to no use to clinical practitioners. Ethicists of all stripes must be both well grounded in the concrete reality of working professionals and experienced enough to have the practical wisdom necessary to assist with real-world problems.

They are wrong in that the skills of philosophical analysis, when combined with instruction in empirical investigation, political awareness, and appropriate character traits, are vital to ethics consulting. That is, ethicists, again of all stripes, need the theoretical and conceptual analysis skills that are a standard part of a philosophical education and mindset, whether acquired through a formal program or self-taught.

I reach this conclusion, admittedly, coming from exactly the sort of background Kass criticizes: I am an academically trained philosopher whose main teaching, writing, and research are in practical ethics. But I reach it also through my experiences working for nearly twenty years as a consulting ethicist, in various capacities at various hospitals. This book emerges, in fact, from those experiences, especially from my early transition into direct clinical consulting and the recognition of some key gaps between how I was trained and the role I was taught to perform and what I discovered the hospital wanted from me.

Having received a doctorate in philosophy with a concentration in bioethics and a certificate in clinical ethics,[6] I enthusiastically jumped at the opportunity to supplement my standard university teaching and research job in a philosophy department by providing a mix of bioethics services for area hospitals—assisting on ethics committees, giving the occasional didactic lecture, and helping in the formulation of policy. The work was gratifying for me and, per the feedback, of real value for them.

Yet my move into more direct clinical consulting was not nearly so successful. The newly appointed director of the area teaching hospital's intensive care unit, fresh from the National Institutes of Health with its extensive ethics programs, realized the residents needed exposure beyond my to-that-point grand rounds–type lectures; they needed direct ethics involvement in clinical cases. He thus invited me to do ethics rounds with his residents. I quickly learned, though, that the very sorts of skills—analytical and theoretical reasoning, problem dissection, connecting key concepts to general ethical concerns—that had served me so well in my previous consulting role were of limited value here. As the director eventually told me in one of those painful but incredibly valuable conversations, "Enough abstractions already. Stop being a philosopher and start being an ethicist. These people need real help with real problems."

After many subsequent conversations about the relative importance of process versus outcomes and of analysis versus action, I agreed to experiment with exactly what I had been trained not to do: I would tell the residents how they should act in these hard cases. Now that can be hedged in a variety of ways—I was only giving recommendations, I was not the final decision maker, I still urged them to rely on their own good moral sense—but in the end, given the consultative structure of hospital culture, especially teaching hospital culture, the reality was I was telling them what to do.

And almost immediately this shift had positive results, exemplified most clearly in that the residents now routinely sought out my help and seemed to genuinely benefit from the advice. As gratifying as all this change was, however, it also created a crisis of conscience. I was, after all, merely a philosopher. I was good at analyzing issues and encouraging the residents to look at problems, and solutions, in different ways, but I was no moral expert. Indeed, it had been adamantly grilled into me throughout my philosophical training that there *was* no such thing. Who was I, or any philosopher, to be telling them the "correct" moral choice?[7]

This book is an attempt to tackle that question. The core thesis is that, assuming a number of crucial caveats, philosopher-ethicists can be moral experts and, again granting caveats, the best persons to provide clinical ethics consulting. The traditional philosophical skills of abstract deliberation and conceptual analysis, combined with the insights gained from studying twenty-five hundred years of ethics theory, provide a method of reasoning that is foundational to the kind of thinking demanded of consulting ethicists on a daily basis.[8]

In drawing this conclusion I reject a principal tenet of what I call the "standard approach" to clinical ethics training and practice. This approach, exemplified in *Core Competencies for Health Care Ethics Consultation* (hereafter, *Core Competencies*),[9] holds that ethicists should restrict their work to ethically facilitating agreement; that is, to analyzing problems, to clarifying concepts and issues, to identifying who and what are at stake in ethical problems, and to helping decision makers reach consensus. Normative elements are clearly present in this approach; for example, the *Core Competencies* urge consultants to "clarify . . . normative issues (e.g., the implications of societal values, law, ethics, and institutional policy for the case)" and to "help to identify a range of morally acceptable options within the context."[10] Missing from the approach, however, is the notion that ethicists should provide direct prescriptive recommendations as to what is the correct moral choice, or at least advice beyond determining which choices fall outside a morally acceptable norm. Instead, the emphasis is clearly on building consensus rather than on prescribing; the consultant's role should be helping to "facilitate the building of morally acceptable shared commitments or understandings within the context."[11] Once moral boundaries are established, the consultant's job is to motivate agreement among the relevant parties within the (potentially quite wide) remaining options. Taking on a more prescriptive role—that is, saying what decision makers *should* do, rather than only saying what they *should not*—is inappropriate, because, the *Core Competencies* aver, there are no ethics experts and because a prescriptive approach too easily slides into authoritarianism.[12]

My contrary thesis—that consultants should sometimes take the normatively positive approach—carries plenty of risk, not the least of which is the implied arrogance. To defend it considerable attention must be paid to what good ethics decision-making entails and why philosophical training makes one well-suited. The structure of the book is hence both a defense of this claim and an explanation of how it can be made plausible. That is, moral expertise demands a range of skills, from ethical reasoning, to political awareness, to a sophisticated empirical methodology.

Thus, like Kass, my position is critical of a fundamental tenet of the standard approach. But because, as noted above, I think that approach gets much right, the book is also intended both as a bridge between those sides and as a kind of guidebook for how to do consulting right. It is not, however, a guidebook for *what* to do in any given ethical problem, the sort of manual one carries in one's white coat, to be whipped out at the bedside. It is not for at least two reasons: First, as I argue in chapters 3 and 4, ethics problems always reside within a political, ideological, and institutional framework. While I think the properly trained philosopher-ethicist, with the right demeanor, is best suited for determining the right answer, each such answer is always context driven. Hence any such manual can be general only, capturing commonalities that regularly recur among such problems. And, second, excellent versions of such generalized guidebooks have been in the field for quite some time, the best of which is *Clinical Ethics*, by Albert Jonsen et al.[13]

This book, instead, gives a meta-analysis of the discipline, directed primarily at academics who teach ethics consulting, and secondarily at current practitioners who might be inclined to acquire tools to do it better. The latter might feel frustrated by the lack of pat answers, but my hope is if they hang in with the arguments—arguments I have striven to make as accessible as possible—those efforts will result in a better understanding of the issues, a better grasp of moral decision-making (and empirical methodology), an enhanced recognition of the impact of political ideology, and, through all this, a greater likelihood of making morally better choices.

The chapters are laid out as follows. In chapter 1 I provide a direct defense of the philosopher-ethicist as moral expert, able to give prescriptive advice in much the same manner as any other clinical consultant. Furthermore, I argue, this is exactly what clinicians seek from ethics consultants: to act as any other consultant would by recommending, as per her best judgment, the most appropriate course of action. There are also caveats aplenty, especially with respect to the need for ethicists to have the right dispositions and character traits.

In chapter 2 I reject Kass's appraisal of the meta- and theoretical foundations that serve as the core to the standard approach.[14] Instead, I defend a method of moral reasoning that synthesizes what I think are the best theoretical approaches, those of Tom Beauchamp and James Childress, Bernard Gert, and virtue theory.

The third and fourth chapters, though, develop and build off another criticism of the standard approach—that it too narrowly regards what is at stake in clinical ethics cases. In chapter 3 I argue that clinical cases are set within political realities, by which I mean two things. The first is the obvious point that clinical ethics problems exist within hospital organizations, each of which has its own institutional politics—its power struggles, turf wars, clearly defined disciplinary hierarchy, and so on. While those politics are often acknowledged and criticized, inadequate attention is given to their impact on, indeed their often being *the cause of*, ethical conflicts.

The second is a more subtle, and ultimately more important, point about social context and political ideologies and how they color the way members of the health care team—clinicians, administrators, and ethicists—perceive and evaluate ethical problems. Too often such problems are treated as if they exist in isolation, disconnected from broader social context. The few exceptions to the general rule, I argue, serve to prove the case. For example, a recognition of economic realities regularly pops up in the common clinical claim that a particular ethical problem would disappear "if only we had adequate funding." But almost never does one hear a similarly politicized comment that, for example, a problem would disappear "if only we did not have such archaic laws regarding same-sex marriages and the legal status of unmarried partners." That is, sticking with the example, it is uncommon in the literature and truly rare for hospital personnel to recognize how an ideological bias against same-sex (or even unmarried heterosexual) partners affects the trust granted to surrogates.

Chapter 3 thus explores the relationship between macrolevel social context and political ideology and microlevel specific cases. Such macro considerations significantly alter how clinical participants perceive ethical issues. This conclusion, I argue, also significantly impacts what count as solutions; that is, truly viable solutions must take the broader context into account. I give a theoretical explanation of the political nature of clinical ethics, provide examples to show how ideology is present in cases, and show ways a politically aware version of ethics consulting would differ. One of the goals here is to reveal that macrolevel beliefs, values, and structures are also present in, and play much the same causal role in, mid-level organizational values, as well as in microlevel clinical decision-making. That is, the structural norms at each of the levels do not exist in isolation of the others but are in fact essentially interconnected.

Key to the argument in chapter 3 is a recognition that individuals' beliefs and values, and thus their choices and actions, emerge from social context. Much of the bioethics literature, by contrast, presents ethics choices as emerging from independent autonomous agents. In chapter 4 I reject that view in some detail. Relying on work especially by Patricia Werhane,[15] I stress the powerful role of the intersubjective organizational mindset or "script,"[16] and discuss its effect on clinical, and ethical, decision-making.

This conclusion, though, also motivates the need for a different empirical method, a different understanding of what facts are important and how to get at them. The heavy reliance on case studies, with factual details typically provided by the physician-in-charge, gets at only a small portion of the important details present in the case and relevant to good clinical ethics decision-making. In addition to such relatively narrow presentations (which usually include relevant medical facts, as these are understood by the presenter, along with varying degrees of reference to "psychosocial" and economic considerations), ethicists also need a sufficiently rich understanding of their particular organizational culture. The ethicist needs to be able to understand the issues as the clinician does, from her perspective. This inside-out view allows the ethicist to better appreciate how institutional agents understand, analyze, and respond to ethical issues. Without that perspective, I argue, ethicist and clinician often talk past one another.

In making these arguments, I characterize the key skills, training, attitude, and political sensibilities of consulting ethicists, thus filling out the "guidebook" purpose noted above, both for individual ethicists and for clinical ethics education programs. In doing this I also try to bring together literature from normally disparate sources, that is, from those who come at these issues from politically moderate, conservative, and leftist perspectives.

My focus is on clinical ethics because that is where most philosophically trained ethicists[17] practice their craft and because it is the arena with which I am most familiar. The arguments, though, carry across professional settings; that is, with minor variants they apply to ethicists working in business, news media, law, government—any context in which organizational structure is complex enough to have an impact on how participants think about and act upon ethical problems. I say this both because my experience in those other settings confirms it[18] and because, as I will argue in chapter 2, the moral foundations that underlie all such settings are the same; that is, while context must be taken into account in any moral analysis, moral norms are not relative to them.

In defining the consultant's appropriate background and training, I hope also to push ethics consulting to the broader discipline's roots, to remind consultants of the macrolevel considerations on which the discipline was founded. Bioethics, since its inception, has had a strong focus on effecting change. Although much of the discipline was concerned mainly with clarifying key concepts and principles (e.g., autonomy, futility, nonmaleficence) and with broad, almost theoretical discussions of specific issues (e.g., abortion, euthanasia, informed consent), there was also a large body of work directly concerned with macrolevel analyses of social and institutional structures. These analyses nearly always had an at least secondary agenda of recommending rearrangements of those structures so as to make them more consistent with general ethical principles, in particular with principles of justice.[19] They also played a critical role in informing debate, especially as such issues as informed consent and patients' right to refuse treatment worked their way through the courts.

This activism strives to analyze moral and social concerns, to make prescriptive recommendations, and to promote structural changes by which these recommendations can best be implemented. I wish, in this book, to extend some of that activist attitude to clinical consulting.

# Notes

1. Andrew Ferguson, "Liberty, Equality, Dignity: Leon Kass Challenges the Scientific Project," *Weekly Standard*, 4 November 2002, 23.

2. Leon R. Kass, *Life, Liberty, and the Defense of Dignity: The Challenge for Bioethics* (San Francisco: Encounter Books, 2002).

3. I would note, however, it is mainly in chapter 2 that Kass is so critical. The remainder of the book is a largely sympathetic, rich, and challenging account of the recent history and current practice of bioethics.

4. Kass, *Life, Liberty*, 57.

5. Barry Hoffmaster, "Can Ethnography Save the Life of Medical Ethics?" *Social Science and Medicine* 35, no. 12 (1992): 1422.

6. The University of Tennessee's program was, at the time (mid-1980s), cutting edge in its mix of traditional philosophical training with extensive clinical exposure.

7. Cf. Rosemary Tong, "The Epistemology and Ethics of Consensus: Uses and Misuses of 'Ethical' Expertise," *Journal of Medicine and Philosophy* 16, no. 4 (August 1991): 409–26; Michael Bayles, "Moral Theory and Application," *Social Theory and*

*Practice* 10, no. 1 (Spring 1984): 97–120; and Arthur Caplan, "Moral Experts and Moral Expertise: Do Either Exist?," in *Clinical Ethics: Theory and Practice*, ed. Barry Hoffmaster, Benjamin Freedman, and Gwen Fraser (Clifton, NJ: Humana Press, 1989), 59–87, especially the A. J. Ayer quotation on page 64.

8. This conclusion also calls into question the "two weeks" movement noted above; that is, a two-week crash course in ethics theory and method cannot provide the philosophical skills requisite to good clinical ethics. Such a course can very well motivate the necessary passion for further study, but it is no substitute for a lifetime commitment to philosophical thinking and reading.

9. *Core Competencies for Health Care Ethics Consultation: The Report of the American Society for Bioethics and Humanities* (Glenville, IL: ASBH, 1998). While much of what follows is a critique of the *Core Competencies*, I consider it to be the most important source for defining the skills, methods, and training best suited for clinical ethics consultation, the sort of document to which all future analyses of clinical ethics must respond.

10. *Core Competencies*, 6.

11. *Core Competencies*, 7.

12. *Core Competencies*, 5–6.

13. Albert Jonsen, Mark Siegler, and William Winslade, *Clinical Ethics*, now in its sixth edition (New York: McGraw-Hill, 2006). See also John LaPuma and David Schiedermayer, *Ethics Consultation: A Practical Guide* (Boston: Jones and Bartlett Publishers, 1994); and Mark Aulisio, Robert Arnold, and Stuart Younger, *Ethics Consultation: From Theory to Practice* (Baltimore, MD: Johns Hopkins University Press, 2003).

14. Kass, *Life, Liberty*, 60.

15. Patricia Werhane, *Moral Imagination and Management Decision-making* (New York: Oxford, 1999).

16. Werhane, *Moral Imagination*, 56.

17. While my arguments concern academically trained philosophers who participate in any of a range of practical ethics consultative activities, for shorthand, except where context demands otherwise, I will use the term "ethicist."

18. This experience includes a total of nearly eight years' combined work as an observer-consultant in local news media, both print and television; one year as a consultant in an ophthalmology clinic; and more than a hundred lectures and workshops for regional government, legal, and business organizations.

19. I have in mind here especially the work of such scholars as Talcott Parsons, Robert Veatch, Howard Waitzken, Ivan Illich, Norman Daniels, Susan Sontag, Allen Buchanan, Eliot Freidson, Edmund Pellegrino, and David Thomasma.

# CHAPTER ONE

~

# Clinical Ethics Consulting and Moral Expertise

What should be the role of clinical ethicists? There is a clear consensus they can and should play an important part in policy development and staff education. There is not, however, similar agreement regarding how case consultations should be handled. Should ethicists merely analyze problems and outline relevant value dimensions? Should they become patient advocates? Physician or hospital advocates? Should they give prescriptive recommendations as to best ethical choices?

The predominant view has long been that the first role—problem analysis—is the most appropriate. This is true both in the literature (as exemplified in the *Core Competencies*) and in practice; for example, the question comes up at least every couple of months on each of the four hospital ethics committees on which I serve, and each time there is overwhelming sentiment that such committees, when fulfilling their consultant role, should stick to the more restricted approach. The reason for this is also widely acknowledged: Our society's respect for a pluralism of values demands it. A related reason is the perceived failure of moral theory; since theorists cannot agree on the philosophical foundations and method for moral decision-making, there are thus no established grounds upon which one could take a stronger approach and give prescriptive advice. Indeed, the seemingly unending and contentious debates in ethics theory have left many skeptical about the value of pursuing right answers in ethics and, even more, about

Significant portions of this chapter were published in my article, "A Defense of the Philosopher-Ethicist as Moral Expert," *The Journal of Clinical Ethics* 14, no. 4 (Winter 2003): 259–69.

whether philosophers have any particular ethics expertise. If philosophers cannot even agree on abstract theory, such skeptics maintain, why on earth should others turn to them for advice when faced with real-world dilemmas? This skepticism has naturally found its way into debates on the ethicist's role, resulting in the standard approach, that of problem analysis.

As noted above, I wish to challenge this standard view and defend, instead, a role that combines good problem analysis with prescriptive recommendations.[1] In doing so I start by assuming that strict relativism in ethics is false. That is, I believe certain basic claims in ethics, for example a prohibition against gratuitous harm,[2] are not only true but also are known with certainty by minimally rational moral agents. I grant, though, that there are not many such obviously true and knowable claims. I grant, also, that to date no moral theory can fully account for these relatively abstract verities while also adequately addressing the mucky realities of moral life. Accepting both these admissions, however, neither undercuts an acceptance of genuine moral truth nor speaks against progress in ethics theory or the importance of philosophical methodology. In other words, that philosophers cannot reach agreement at the level of theory does not mean the standard philosophical repertoire of deductive and inductive reasoning, arguments by analogy, use of metaphors and narratives, appeals to intuition, and so on, cannot get us to, or at least *closer to*, moral truth. To deny the value of this method is also to deny what philosophers routinely teach in our introduction and logic courses—namely, that careful reasoned analysis is vital to intellectual pursuits and the search for truth. Thus, to deny that same methodological value within a clinical setting is cynical at best, philosophical obstinacy at worst.

From this admittedly controversial starting point, one I assume here and do not defend, I will argue that ethicists can and should adopt some version of the role of the "moral expert" in clinical settings, since, assuming crucial caveats detailed below, they are typically in a better position to get at least closer to moral truth than are their clinical counterparts. In defending this conclusion I briefly critique the two main competing positions. I also describe what I think are the skills and attitudes that best promote effective, morally sound, and institutionally sensitive ethics consulting, with such skills (and likely also such attitudes) being significant additions to philosophers' standard training and skills.

## Moral Expertise

Even many of the bioethicists who have accepted the standard view have also taken considerable pride from the impact that philosophically grounded bioethics, combined with the work of patient advocates and legal activists, has had in altering medical practice. In the last thirty years alone, far greater emphasis has been placed, for example, on enhancing informed consent requirements, promoting confidentiality, shifting the medical culture away from paternalism and toward autonomy, creating greater protections for research subjects, enhancing the rights of children to have more of a voice in their medical care, and, maybe most importantly if not always with complete success, reinforcing respect for patients as whole persons rather than as mere physical specimens. That is, bioethicists accept that, in these respects at least, health care is a morally better environment than it was prior to the bioethics movement.

Despite this pride, however, the literature at the same time overwhelmingly rejects a similar role for microlevel, case-based clinical consulting. The clinical ethicist's job, as it is typically conceived, is not to promote what she personally believes to be the morally best choice, or at least not beyond the value of respecting the rights of decision makers and the democratic, consensus-building such respect promotes. Rather, her job is merely to assist practitioners to better understand what is morally at stake, including general moral boundaries, and then to help facilitate consensual agreement among conflicted parties. These two outcomes, the standard approach avers, help create an environment in which specific better moral outcomes may emerge, but whether they do is secondary to other *process*-based considerations, especially the extent to which agreement is facilitated.

This need not be seen as an endorsement of moral relativism (though I think it often is, given the history and sociology of the discipline of philosophy, as I show below); one could remain silent on that question theoretically but take a pragmatic, or epistemologically skeptical, stance relative to hard, real-world ethical problems. That is, one could embrace even the best consultants' inability to grasp moral truth when immersed in all the messy details clinical ethics cases bring with them, and pragmatically rely upon the more limited truth that, generally speaking, persons' voices should be heard. This is, as I interpret it, the position of the *Core Competencies*, and it is reinforced by Mark Aulisio and Robert Arnold (among the principal authors of the *Core Competencies*) in response to an earlier version of this argument:

Approximating moral truth . . . should not be the goal of ethics consultation. There is a deep sense in which, on our view, "moral truth" is irrelevant for ethics consultation. This is largely due to the fact that issues which arise in the clinic emerge in a context in which individuals retain their political rights to live according to their own moral views, even if those views turn out to be false from some other particular moral point of view—even, per hypothesis, the "correct moral view." We suggest that there is a deep sense in which clinical ethics consultation is more in the domain of the political than the moral, and more in the domain of practice than theory. Given its context, the appropriate question for ethics consultation is most often "Who should be allowed to decide?" rather than "Which view most approximates moral truth?"[3]

The whole paragraph has pragmatic overtones, as exemplified in their two uses of the term "political."[4] The first usage is in relation to "rights" and serves to confine this key moral concept to a *civil*, rather than a *moral* or *natural*, status. The latter, moral/natural conception of rights is normatively much richer in that it applies to all persons as such; by contrast, Aulisio and Arnold's qualifier restricts rights to only those civil systems that explicitly acknowledge their status. Their second usage of "political" suggests the need to reach compromise and to build agreement within the politics of institutional settings, an approach of course wholly consistent with the consensus model the *Core Competencies* generally recommend. Again, though, this need not be read as a relativist or amoral position, but its normativity is quite narrow, in that value is attached only to autonomy, that is, the right "to live according to their own moral views, even if those views turn out to be false from, . . . per hypothesis, the 'correct moral view.'"

My approach, by contrast, sees autonomy as *one* of many important moral considerations. In fact, placing so much emphasis here can actually be a way of *avoiding* moral commitment. Since we are unwilling—for pragmatic or theoretical reasons—to declare our moral point of view (more) correct, we instead take the morally tolerant position, respecting all participants' autonomous choices. That is, since on the facilitation model moral truth is at best a suspect notion, and since this results in a corresponding insistence upon respect for moral pluralism, the moral goal for ethics consultants is not to seek what they take to be the right choice, but instead to make sure everyone's voice is appropriately heard, even if the consultant strongly believes the resulting actions are morally wrong. The emphasis is almost wholly on process, rather than on strongly promoting the position the consultant believes morally correct.

While such promotion of democratic, autonomous processes is undoubtedly of great moral worth, it is not the only value present in clinical ethics decision-making, nor should it always trump all other values, including beneficence and justice. I say this in part because, in practice, patient autonomy is such an elusive goal, particularly in end-of-life choices.[5] It is elusive because of illness, fear, pain, patients' socialization, and, as I will argue more fully below, because power too often prevails, even when the discussion structure is conscientiously designed to promote individual autonomy and genuinely democratic processes. Further, surely it is preferable to combine both, that is, to have a process that respects and encourages participation *and* that gets as close as possible to the right answer.

That latter goal obviously requires a kind of moral expertise well beyond that of promoting autonomy-driven consensus. This more extensive version of normativity seeks to judge among the multiple values at stake, including autonomy, and to urge the one that gets closest to truth.

## The Rejection of Truth

As noted, the reluctance to see normativity and the consultant's role in this richer sense is hardly unique to Aulisio and Arnold. It is, rather, the standard view, one grounded in important social and historical roots. Western culture, with its varied religious and political perspectives, has persistently attempted to promote a commitment to tolerance, while at the same time struggling over its appropriate limits. This commitment, though, too often spills over into a kind of schizophrenic moral relativism, schizophrenic because of the often simultaneous appeals to tolerance and to unhesitating moral condemnation of perceived evil. Consider, for example, what will be the near-universal reaction, in the United States at least, to the eventual capture or killing of Osama Bin Laden.

Philosophy has also long grappled with this tension and settled on a pretty broad consensus of relativism in the Anglo-American philosophy of the mid-1950s, with its pervasive rejection of normative ethics. Art Caplan makes a similar tracing, quoting A. J. Ayer's particularly blunt rejection:

> It is silly, as well as presumptuous, for any one type of philosopher to pose as the champion of virtue. And it is also one reason why many people find moral philosophy an unsatisfying subject. For they mistakenly look to the moral philosopher for guidance.[6]

While Ayer's comments might be dismissed as reflective of the then-dominant logical positivism he helped promote, they are closely matched by Michael Bayles's more recent observations:

> It is ludicrous for a hospital to have an ethicist on a beeper for call to the bedside to make instant thumbs up or thumbs down decisions. The work of ethics involves careful and detailed analysis and reflection, precisely what is not possible in the practical world. Hence, while ethicists can sometimes handle hard cases better than practitioners, their relative strength is not at the level of

action. Rather the role of applied ethics is to reflect upon such situations and help practitioners be clearer about what to look for and how much weight to assign to considerations when they must make decisions. Ethicists are not specialists on a par with perinatologists, tax lawyers, and structural engineers.[7]

These sorts of criticisms have definitely stuck; very few writers are willing to defend the philosopher-as-expert view, and even when they do, it is usually presented in one of two weakened forms, neither of which has much connection with seeking moral truth—that is, philosopher-ethicists are merely experts at either problem analysis or at achieving consensus.[8]

## Experts in Analysis

The approach of the first such weakened form is to substantially narrow the scope of expertise, as captured in the following characteristic comment by Rosemary Tong in her discussion of the role of ethics committees:

> Even if all the members of an ethics committee had formal training in ethical reasoning, only their *procedural* skills as professional ethicists—and not also their *substantive* conclusions as moral agents—could be non-problematically offered to other moral agents. Ethics is not a set of conclusions that experts pass on to non-experts; rather, it is a set of decision-making tools that non-experts as well as experts must use if they are to reach their own conclusions about what is morally permitted, required, or forbidden to them. . . . Morality is a *personal* quest.[9]

Any expertise philosophers might bring to the table, she thus concludes, exists only in their particular strengths at problem analysis, at figuring out what is at stake in moral problems—who will be affected, what values (or principles or rules) are involved, what are likely consequences—and using these to help practitioners reach their own "personal" (i.e., autonomous) conclusions regarding the morally best choice.

Tong is right that well-trained philosophers are especially skilled at such analysis and thus can provide real assistance in getting at the heart of ethics problems. As noted above, however, these skills emerge from the standard philosophical methodology of deduction, induction, intuition, and empirical examination. And this method is of course not arbitrarily chosen—philosophers rely on it precisely because they believe reasoned scrutiny gives us *better, more accurate* answers. Put another way, philosophers rely upon rational analysis for good reason—because they believe it can get them at least closer to the truth of the matter in these difficult moral dilemmas.

Some writers have in fact argued for an outright rejection of even Tong's recommended approach, urging instead methods grounded in group psychology and political management that are intended merely to promote, or "facilitate,"[10] agreement among conflicted parties. I will critique this position in depth below. My argument here is there is a natural progression from Tong's conclusion that philosophical analysis gets closer to the truth of the *problem* to mine that the same method also gets closer to the truth of the *answer*. In short, my conclusion is that the ethicist should be an advocate, but not for the patient, or the physician or the hospital. Rather, she advocates the best ethical outcome.[11]

Five arguments reveal this progression from analyst to advocate. First, there is the implication in Tong's argument that the sorts of "procedural skills" to which she refers are themselves nonnormative, that philosopher-ethicists can provide *objective* analyses of problems, of what and who are at stake. But surely this is false. Any analysis of a problem comes with a normative underpinning. The very determination of the "stakes" is an explicitly normative enterprise, since it assigns value to some concerns, and to some people, rather than to others. Upon what theoretical foundations and ethical biases are such judgments based and how is the analysis of the problem being affected? That such foundations and biases are often not transparent, even to the person holding them, does not mean they are not present. Indeed, beliefs without an ethically informed foundation would be far worse, little better than ad hoc reactions to empirical information. Bernard Gert puts it even more bluntly. In his defense of a rational and impartial morality he says, "To deny the systematic nature of morality is to deny that applied and professional ethics is an academic discipline."[12] Is it not both more honest and more rational to acknowledge a point of view and to give reasoned arguments in support of corresponding prescriptive recommendations?

Second, recall Bayles's words quoted above: "It is ludicrous for a hospital to have an ethicist on a beeper for call to the bedside to make instant thumbs up or thumbs down decisions. The work of ethics involves careful and detailed analysis and reflection, precisely what is not possible in the practical world." But why is it any more "ludicrous" for an ethicist, a person whose professional life is devoted to the study and practice of moral theory and decision-making, to make these decisions than for a clinician to do so? Better to leave it to the medical resident in the midst of a thirty-six-hour shift, or to the terribly overworked nurse buried in paperwork, or to the attending physician trying to juggle patient care, resident education, three committee meetings, and various other institutional pressures and constraints? Even the moral skeptic must acknowledge that the ethicist can hardly do worse than harried clinicians, and generally will do better, assuming she brings appropriate attitudes and skills, as discussed below.

Third, some critics, though, contend that good clinical ethics decisions demand *experience*.[13] While this is undoubtedly true, hospital ethicists often have far more extensive experience, particularly with the kinds of difficult cases on which they would be called, than have residents and young attending staff. Also, the kind of experience required is of conflicting *values*, and thus is attainable from multiple sources. One of the mistakes clinicians, even the most experienced, often make is to see medical judgments as value-free, as being only about "objective" medicine. The ethicist can help break through that false objectivity, revealing the range of values present in the case. For this, her experience as an *ethicist*, rather than any experience one might bring as a clinician, is what is vital.

Fourth, the consultant as expert is more consistent with the medical ethos, with its ever-narrowing specialization and concomitant attachment of expertise. This is especially true in the teaching hospital environment, where medical students and residents are explicitly trained to seek the help of expert specialists. Such practitioners demand more than mere problem analysis, and rightly so. To provide a rich, complex analysis of a problem—determining what conceptual problems are present and what principles or virtues are at stake, evaluating consequences and their ethical implications—and then to avoid making an actual recommendation seems to many of those working in the trenches as at best awkward and incomplete. Indeed, it often makes the clinicians' eventual decision-making all the more difficult, at least in those cases that involve genuine moral dilemmas (and not just confusion over facts). The ethicist takes a problem with which clinicians are already struggling and then, through her analysis, reveals just how complex and difficult it is. Then she leaves? Some help that is.

Last, the approach is also dishonest, since the ethicist almost assuredly has reached an opinion on the case and, knowingly or otherwise, subtly communicates that opinion in her case analysis. Better, therefore, to be up front and give a recommendation, tempered of course by appropriate caveats about one's own ethical biases and background, and justified with good philosophical reasoning. Clinicians are explicitly taught to reflect critically upon expert advice and to use the process as an opportunity to learn, steps they should of course also take with any ethics advice. But imagine a resident's distress at calling for a cardiology consultation, only to have the specialist arrive, engage in sophisticated problem analysis, and then depart without having given any advice as to how to help cure the ailment. While the analogy to ethics consulting is not precise,[14] it is close enough to again reveal how odd is the strict problem-analysis model.

## Justified Reasons and Consensus

The second weakened version of ethics expertise prevalent in the literature gives up, or at least sidesteps, the search for genuine moral truth, and instead seeks only justified reasons for making moral claims as grounded in social consensus or coherentist views.[15] I will give a brief description of two different versions, with arguments for why I believe each to be inadequate.

The first consensus model emerges from Jurgen Habermas's public discourse ethics. David Casarett et al. do an admirable job of summarizing Habermas's notoriously difficult arguments: Because reality, including its moral components, is intersubjectively determined, they argue, the best persons can hope for is consensus over its nature, achieved through discourse-based dispute and discussion. As Casarett et al. put it, because of the intersubjectively constituted nature of reality, "In the end, public communication, rather than private deduction, becomes the method by which validity is established."[16] For it—validity—truly to be achieved, however, *full* agreement must be present. Habermas's version of Kant's universalization principle requires that "*all* affected can accept the consequences and side effects its general observance can be expected to have for the satisfaction of *everyone's* interests."[17] While the approach admits of a kind of relativism, at least of one with respect to absolute truth, its intersubjectivity (combined with a series of constraints on how the discourse, as rational, should proceed), they claim, at least prevents it from being a *radical* relativism.[18]

Consensus building is undoubtedly an important function of clinical ethics case consultations. As the *Core Competencies* aver, the morally correct course of action in any given clinical situation must represent the complex interplay of patient preferences, legal rights, and professional standards, as these are determined through a careful process devoted to achieving group agreement.[19] It is important but in the end inadequate, for two reasons. First, it appeals to, indeed it *assumes*, moral relativism, and as such runs contrary to my opening assumptions.

Second, and more importantly, even if one grants some form of relativism, the consensualist's aim of achieving full agreement cannot be accomplished in clinical ethics practice. Even with a careful and carefully structured discourse process—Casarett et al. describe the Habermasian ethicist's job as "gathering data, enhancing communication, identifying areas of ethical discomfort, and clarifying the goals of participants," all with the aim of ensuring "that everyone who would be affected by a decision is able to participate"[20]—there is still insufficient attention paid to the impact of *power* within discourse. Those who hold power, especially power historically established within a hierarchical institution like medicine, characteristically dominate conversations. They control the tone, they control the content, and they usually control the outcomes. To believe that ethicists can substantially alter those power dynamics is simply naive.[21]

To illustrate, I have worked for nearly twenty years at four hospitals in my community and am well established in all of them in my role as clinical ethicist, particularly at the teaching hospital. I also am a tenured, full professor of philosophy, have a clinical certificate in bioethics, run an ethics center, have been a long-term department chair, and am regularly called upon for public comment and advice on current ethical issues. Furthermore, I am also a physically large, white male with a deep voice and a goodly amount of self-confidence. In other words, I am just the sort of person who in normal discourse has at least equal, if not dominant, power. Yet in the rigidly hierarchical world of institutional medicine, even I routinely have to struggle to be heard when the group is dominated by physicians, especially those from such specialties as cardiology, neurology, and surgery. Imagine, thus, the difficulties faced by typically female and often nonwhite nurses, ancillary clinical staff, social workers, and the like. And the persons who most need to be heard in these conversations—patients and families—are usually by far the most intimidated. These dynamics are deeply entrenched in institutional and social cultures and pervade in ways of which even the participants in conversations are often unaware.[22] Thus the discourse-based consensus sought by Habermas/Casarett et al. is unrealistic. Or, better, a type of verbal consensus may well emerge, but it will *only* be verbal—that is, there will be a disconnect between what has been verbally agreed to and what actions are taken—and thus nothing close to Habermas's idealized goal.

## Coherence

The second model builds upon a promising theory of moral epistemology,[23] coherentism, first developed by John Rawls[24] and later elaborated on by Norman Daniels (who dubs its idealized form "wide reflective equilibrium" [hereafter WRE]).[25] In simple terms, the method seeks coherence among all normatively related beliefs; that is, it engages a process whereby the various layers of moral reasoning—specific judgments, prescriptive rules or principles, empirical claims about facts of the world, and background theory—are brought into equilibrium. One starts with moral judgments about which one feels very confident (Rawls gives religious intolerance and racial discrimination as examples[26]) and then balances these confidently held judgments against rules or principles, factual beliefs, and relevant scientific and normative theories, all with the goal of achieving a coherent fit.[27] In this balancing, furthermore, one will frequently have to make adjustments at each of the levels, even, occasionally, to the initial intuitive judgments.[28]

The value of a WRE approach, Rawls and Daniels argue, is that it avoids sticky and potentially irresolvable foundationalist, metaphysical, and epistemological questions about the nature of reality and its epistemological accessibility. In so avoiding, Rawls and Daniels also remain agnostic on the question of whether such coherence gets at moral *truth*. As Daniels describes it, if there is such a thing as moral truth, WRE provides the best method for getting at it; if not, it is the best alternative available as it at least gives us objective *reasons*.[29] Thus as Scott Yoder concludes (as he recommends WRE as a method for applied ethics), "[E]xpertise in ethics is not dependent on the existence of objective moral knowledge. . . . The key is to see that [such] expertise . . . is connected with *justification*—a claim to ethics expertise is not based on the truth of one's judgments, but on one's ability to provide a coherent justification for them."[30]

Coherentism has been recommended as an applied ethics methodology from two angles. The first is for the ethicist to use WRE to develop her own coherent set of beliefs and then use these to justify her clinical analyses and recommendations. This approach is currently among the most popular in applied ethics[31] and certainly is consistent with my call for clinical ethicists to rely on standard philosophical methods of analytic reasoning; WRE is clearly a powerful (and possibly truth-getting) tool of ethics reasoning and thus is also wholly compatible with my recommended approach. While I am deeply skeptical that one could ever achieve complete equilibrium—there are too many beliefs, values, and scientific theories to be brought into alignment—there is nonetheless considerable value in the ongoing self-reflective analysis commitment to the approach entails. That is, the approach attempts to bring to fruition Socrates' famous dictum to "know thyself," including thy beliefs, values, and theories.

The second approach is even less practical—achieving coherence among all participants' beliefs, judgments, and so forth. Done correctly, this kind of coherence would necessarily also produce consensus, since all participants would agree on relevant decisional factors.

Achieving coherence among one's beliefs, judgments, principles, and theories is tough enough; to achieve this also for all participants in a decision really is nigh on impossible. Because of this, such coherentism in practice merges into a consensualist model of the sort criticized above. Ironically, Daniels himself gives an example of this in his essay, "Wide Reflective Equilibrium in Practice."[32] After describing the method in theoretical terms, Daniels discusses a case in which he believes it was effectively used, when he was a part of a "diverse group of academics . . . [with] diverse . . . philosophical training and beliefs," working together to develop a set of principles and values to underlie the Clinton administration's health care reform proposal.[33] The group was successful, he says, because it was "able to *agree* on some fourteen basic 'principles and values' that we thought ought to govern health care reform."[34] Missing from his description, however, is any discussion of a *coherent* melding of what must have been conflict among participants' preexisting moral judgments, beliefs, principles, and so forth. Given the acknowledged diverse training and beliefs, achieving true WRE among them would certainly be an onerous task of extensive logical reasoning devoted to discovering and amending inevitable inconsistencies. While that may have taken place, it certainly seems odd that Daniels would not trumpet the process, given that he uses the case as an example of WRE at work. In fact, the much stronger suggestion is that the group merely worked together to reach an agreed upon compromise, one all could live with so as to present a united, *consensus-based* front to the administration and its critics. Granted, achieving such consensus is an impressive feat. It is not, however, an example of WRE at work. Rather, if my reading is accurate, Daniels's example represents a variant on the consensualist approach described above and is thus vulnerable to the same criticisms.[35]

Daniels does go on to describe three other cases and notes his great surprise at finding how his beliefs, primarily at the level of judgment rather than at that of principle, were altered as he worked through the problems and listened to others' arguments.[36] While his description of what motivates those belief alterations bears resemblance to what would be involved in a WRE process, it is not, or at least his description of it is not, anything close to a complete version, since he describes only his own and not other committee members' changes and since those changes occur only at the level of judgment. If anything, his description reads much more like a fairly typical example of being shown that one's judgments cannot be reasonably sustained by one's principles and theory.

As noted, the value of collaborative discussion in applied ethics reasoning and consulting hardly need be defended; my recommended model, as will become more apparent in the attitude and skills section below, is scarcely that of the Lone Ranger ethicist, acting independently of others' advice and contributions.[37] Part of the collaborative value emerges from the attempt to achieve at least relatively narrow reflective coherency among participants' conflicting beliefs and judgments, and this is, in fact, one of the ways that (socially sensitive) philosophers' expertise in critical thinking can be put to best use. But the reality of clinical ethics disputes involving various participants is such that genuinely wide reflective equilibrium among all parties' multilevel moral beliefs and judgments is, again, not possible, for a range of reasons. There are obvious time constraints. There are also complex social constraints since no one, and particularly not authoritative attending physicians, especially appreciates the coldly logical philosopher making apparent one's multilevel moral inconsistencies. Sensitively done, however, such critical thinking skills can better achieve a more logically coherent consensus and can thereby better facilitate and mediate among conflicted parties. But, for all the reasons noted above, one should not pretend any of this would result in either a truly justifying WRE or a Habermasian idealized consensus.

## Attitude and Skills

Some readers by now probably have an image of the ethicist gliding through hospital corridors, halo firmly established, stopping occasionally to bless patients and staff with ethical truth. My vision is anything but. Rather, I believe we do far better to recall the humility urged by Annette Baier when she asks, "Should we not, at least occasionally, . . . consider why the rest of society should not merely tolerate but subsidize our [philosophers'] activity?" followed by the facetious query, "Social conditions have recently changed enough to make philosophers welcome in hospitals, playing there a role once played, approximately, by chaplains. Are we the new priesthood?"[38]

Just because I believe philosophical methods can lead to moral truth does not mean I also believe that any given philosopher-ethicist holds that truth. The best most of us can hope for is to get *closer*, and then only if we recognize our own shortcomings enough to be extraordinarily diligent, thorough, careful, and open-minded.

One of the tougher obstacles philosophers face is moving from emotionally absent abstraction to real cases, with real people, real costs, and real pain. Most philosophers are trained in a manner such that even when cases are used, they are broadly abstract and usually fictional. And when real, the people and circumstances involved are so far removed—temporally, geographically, and culturally—the inclination is still to treat them as merely theoretical, rather than as *humanly real*. Thus there is a tendency to carry that same abstraction into the hospital setting, to forget that any advice we give has the potential for profound impact on actual people's lives. Keeping that impact clearly in mind, though, is vital to reinforcing a requisite sense of awesome responsibility and concomitant diligent care. Consulting ethicists should therefore take seriously Sidney Callahan's conclusion that

[e]xcellent ethical judgment, or better yet, ethical discernment, demands personal moral wisdom and an ardent commitment to seek the true and the good,

[all present in a] good person, . . . [one who possesses] emotional literacy, mature self-discipline, cultivated interpersonal sympathies, and a steadfast personal commitment to high moral standards of worth.[39]

Callahan has set an appropriately high measure, one that should elicit both
humility and a recognition of the monumental burden that comes with making recommendations that, often as not in ethics consulting, help determine
whether a patient lives or dies. Commitment to this attitude also serves to
blunt the criticism sometimes levied against the moral expert view—that it
is antidemocratic since it assigns expertise in an area, moral decision-making,
normally taken to demand tolerant pluralism.[40] One response to this criticism has been voiced by Caplan and seems clearly right. Guarding against
antidemocratic paternalism, he notes, does not mean "wise and prudent persons should not heed the advice of experts on a variety of subjects, including
ethics, in deciding how to live or behave."[41] Furthermore, acknowledging
such expertise, he says, need not thereby create "an elite of moral experts
who have the authority to impose their judgments on others."[42] I know of no
hospital that *requires* that an ethicist be consulted, let alone that her recommendations be followed.[43] No antidemocratic authority is granted the ethicist; to the contrary, as noted above, most ethicists struggle even to establish
a potent position within the hospital hierarchy.

Second, Callahan's recommended humility speaks forcefully against any
antidemocratic arrogance. The conscientious ethicist realizes she is there
only to provide help, help sought by persons in emotional distress, with life-
altering consequences likely attached to accepted advice. If anything, a genuine realization of this staggering responsibility and the careful and deliber-
ate work required not to create havoc in people's lives, should undercut any
temptation toward power-seeking authoritarianism.

Furthermore, the vast majority of clinical ethicists also have an educational role within the institution, certainly education of residents and medical students, often of attending physicians and other professionals (nursing,
social work, etc.), and occasionally of patients and families. When clinical
ethicists do their jobs well, they teach others to make better informed, more
philosophically grounded decisions on their own, thereby again undercutting
an exclusively authoritative role for the ethicist. Indeed, as one clinical col-
league recently put it, my best possible success in my clinical ethics work
would achieve the opposite effect: that is, rather than granting antidemocratic authority, it would instead make me less vital because by effectively edu-
cating others, I reduce their reliance upon my skills.

## Training

Attitude, alone, of course, is not sufficient, as there is also a need for more technical expertise, based in trained skills. I take for granted that anyone wishing to be a philosopher-ethicist will have received extensive post-baccalaureate training in philosophy with an emphasis in theoretical and applied ethics. The ethicist also needs an array of other intellectual and interpersonal skills:[44]

- As noted, experience is critical, both of the clinical environment and of a wide range of other professional, business, and interpersonal contexts. In some sense this is a catch-22: How can a philosopher-ethicist gain clinical experience unless she is a consultant within that setting? The solution is twofold—graduate-level training must include clinical work,[45] and, once employed, the consulting ethicist should commit to extensive immersion in her specific clinical environment, since each brings its own cultural norms, a point on which I will elaborate in chapter 4. Furthermore, until she gains the necessary experience, the ethicist should opt for a reduced, less prescriptive role.
- The ethicist must be able to sufficiently appreciate cases' emotional and personal elements, as opposed to being concerned only with conceptual or theoretical issues. As Tong puts it, "[A]bstract thought, detached from faces and real-life situations, depersonalizes all involved. . . . [Consultants] must be careful lest their attempt to be impartial makes them treat people as equal, faceless, interchangeable atoms in the universe."[46] As noted above, one of bioethicists' harshest critiques of medicine has been its propensity to depersonalize patients. Surely we should take that same concern to heart. A case can be made that many people enter academic life exactly to escape into a life of the mind, avoiding the emotional turmoils of the real world. Given the often disturbing reality of the clinical environment, exacerbated by the fact that ethicists are called for only the most difficult (and thus emotionally traumatic) cases, such reality-avoiding academics should not become consulting ethicists. And for those who do become consulting ethicists, one method of avoiding the, I think, inevitable self-protective tendency to depersonalize is to go regularly to the bedside, engaging the patient and family, seeing real humans with their real struggles and pain.
- Although the clinical ethicist must be careful to avoid becoming a legal consultant, she needs to have familiarity with major bioethics court rulings and legislation. I cannot count the number of times I have

heard a physician exclaim, "I cannot remove the feeding tube! That's illegal!" Simple reassurance that, in appropriate circumstances, such an action is indeed legal often does the trick, but every now and then it becomes necessary to be able to cite relevant case law or legislation. The physician may still refuse—to stick with the example—to withdraw nutrition, but she must now at least give *ethical* as opposed to *legal* reasons. And, in my experience, once the legal threat is removed, many otherwise reluctant physicians will readily consider a much broader range of treatment options.

- For the reasons noted above, the kinds of critical thinking, conceptual framing, and argument analysis skills described by Tong are obviously vital. The ethicist must also be quick on her feet, succinct, and able to use moral imagination[47] to see relationships among problems. Very few physicians (or nurses) have the time or patience for philosophers' normally long, and long-winded, reflective thought and argument.

- Communication is key to most of applied ethics, and is especially so in the current specialized health care environment. Many ethical dilemmas emerge because one medical service is not clear about another's treatment plan, let alone about what has been communicated to patients or family. Add to this the heavy ego involvement many physicians bring, along with the emotional turmoil felt by patients, family, and clinical staff, and the ethicist must be particularly skilled at enhancing and mediating effective dialogue.[48] Furthermore, the better the ethicist is at her job, the more staff will rely upon her to lead the conversation. Yet, most philosophers are not particularly trained in communication skills. Hence those wishing to undertake ethics consulting will need to pay particular attention to acquiring such facility.

- Medical organizations are rigidly structured hierarchical institutions, with clearly established pecking orders. The ethicist must therefore be politically savvy, able to discern that structure, and skilled at interacting accordingly. For example, language that would be effective with, indeed is expected by, a second-year resident would be deeply offensive to a well-established attending physician. I will elaborate on the political nature of hospital organizations, and the necessary concomitant skills for good ethics consulting, in chapter 3.

- Although many of these noted skills involve traditional philosophical activities, others depend on a sophisticated understanding of the empirical facts. Such facts include not just those of the specific case being discussed but also those of the institutional environment, even the professional culture. Literature in business ethics now almost universally accepts that organizational cultures deeply influence the nature of ethical problems and individuals' response to them.[49] Yet most clinical ethicists seem content to rely upon the case study method that has dominated the field, settling for a fairly limited range of facts, typically provided by the physician or other clinician. Because such case presentations generally do not include a description and evaluation of organizational culture and its impact on the case, there is often a problematic gap between what clinicians take to be important and what viable options are, and what ethicists similarly conclude. This is the central point of chapter 4, but the shorthand answer for now is that ethicists should acquire different methods for attaining and understanding the empirical setting in which they work, methods that reveal the organizational culture and ethos.

Chapters 3 and 4 also stress that cases will always be context dependent; ideological and organizational factors present in the institutional setting play a large part in defining the nature of the problem, making generalizations difficult. Nonetheless it may be helpful to show, through a case analysis, how my approach differs from the traditional. One of the hospitals at which I consult received a patient with severe head and abdominal injuries after being struck by a truck. All the injuries were survivable, but after sufficient time passed, everyone agreed that because of the severe head trauma he was now in a permanent vegetative state. He was, however, homeless and a diligent search found no family or close friends. One of the members of the ethics committee requested a consult to discuss whether withdrawal of care was appropriate.

This request alone produced an indignant response from the trauma/surgery team managing the patient, indignant because they, mistakenly, believed it would clearly be illegal to withdraw care and because this service has long been adamant about retaining control of its patients. Institutional policy allowed, however, any member of the hospital staff to request a consult and so eight of us gathered—a representative from the trauma/surgery team, the medical director, the ICU director, the inpatient/nursing service director, the risk manager, the chair of the patients' rights committee, the ethics committee chair (a family practice physician), and myself. (The hospital attorney, unable to attend, had been consulted prior to the meeting and confirmed that while the law was unsettled on these kinds of cases, there was no clear legal impediment against withdrawing care, assuming a genuinely diligent search.) In short, the group brought a nice mix of different services and perspectives, just the sort the consensus model would recommend.

On the traditional model, my job would be to help clarify the values at stake (e.g., quality of life, physician authority and boundaries, nonmaleficence, and substituted autonomy), to make sure everyone's voice was respectfully heard, and, if possible, to try to get all the parties to agree on the best course of action. My own moral judgment would not be of particular relevance, at least not beyond one more alternative to consider.

In reality, of the four physicians, three were male and the fourth, the ICU director, was not only female but had been a resident at the hospital a few years prior (and thus was still trying to establish authority). The remaining participants, other than me, were women and, of course, nonphysicians. From the outset, the surgeon used his position, an aggressive demeanor, and his hospital status—that is, his *power*—to intimidate other participants. He made it clear he was there only because he had to be; no matter what we said, his and the team's minds were made up. As an outsider with less personally at stake,[50] I could and did strive to let others voice their opinions, but none were willing to challenge him directly, especially since the medical director, also a surgeon, was deferring to him. The conversation clearly did not represent anything close to a Habermasian ideal of equal voices, but it *did* represent a common reality in this and most hospitals. Again, on the traditional model, my task would have been to analyze the problem and do all I could to facilitate agreement. And the surgeon would have walked away, secure in the rightness of his position, with no one having strongly taken an opposing view.

Instead, I pushed him on a number of inconsistencies in his argument, mainly having to do with his own judgment about a minimally acceptable quality of life and his admission that should *any* legal relative, even the most remote, show up and request withdrawal, he would happily abide by that decision. I also strongly expressed my own moral judgment, using intentionally harsh language like "condemning this poor man to a life without living." In other words, I strongly *advocated* for a position, rather than just analyzing and facilitating. While I did not succeed in changing his position in this case, I did alter the dynamics of this and future conversations and also, I was later told, convinced others there may be appropriate circumstances in which hospital staff may use substituted judgment and withdraw care.

This is, admittedly, a scary prospect. Who am I to make (or urge) life-or-death decisions for others? To repeat my earlier comment, it is certainly no scarier than leaving such choices to, in this case, a physician driven, I am convinced, mainly by fear of litigation and by his departmental culture.[51]

# Conclusion

From all this emerges my understanding of what "ethics expertise" entails. The analytic, conceptual, and theoretical skills discussed by Tong serve as the intellectual core, but they clearly must be supplemented by experience-based moral wisdom; the ability to listen with care and discernment; the ability to speak and write with clarity and precision; skill at managing egos, emotions, and political environments so as best to facilitate effective communication; sufficient understanding of one's own hierarchy of values; and knowledge of one's limitations. Aulisio and Arnold argue that some of these skills—namely "facilitation," "mediation," and the management of institutional politics—are distinct from seeking truth in ethics.[52] While that argument is consistent with the standard view, and probably also consistent with most of the tradition in philosophical ethics, my argument throughout this book is that all these skills make up expertise in ethics and thus the best prepared ethics consultants will have facility in all.

And, thus, by this point one has to wonder why on earth anyone would take on ethics consulting. If my arguments are right, the training and skills required for clinical ethics are extensive and the attitude is humbling. While to some extent the picture I have drawn is of an ideal, I do want to stress that this is (or should be) very consuming work, in time, energy, and emotions. The ethicist's advice is generally sought only in the truly difficult cases, the ones that are not just ethically complex, but emotionally disturbing. While there can be a range of direct rewards—for example, improved teaching through using one's experiences to translate the merely abstract into the real, rich sources for potential scholarship, financial compensation, and the satisfaction attached to using philosophical training directly to improve patients' lives—there is also a great demand upon one's professional energy, energy that might otherwise go into publications or teaching.[53]

Yet, if the literature is an accurate reflection, many philosophers seem to believe that because they are well trained in ethics theory and critical thinking they should be able to just walk into the clinical environment and immediately be of help. Depending on background, experience, and personality, this may be true, but there is also the potential to cause great harm. Clinicians, especially residents and interns, are truly seeking advice and will likely in fact do what we recommend. Thus it would seem we have an obligation to be as well-prepared, as skilled, and as conscientious as possible. The following chapters thus detail what I take to be the critical skills—ethics reasoning, political and ideological awareness, and realizing the impact of organizational culture.

# Notes

1. "Prescriptive" is clearly a loaded term, one possibly suggesting a more auto-cratic role than I defend. I use it mainly for stylistic reasons, given that the closer in-tent—something like "normatively persuasive"—is awkward at best.

2. Lou Hodges gives a disturbing but nonetheless effective version of this princi-ple, namely, "sandpapering the eyeballs of a three-year-old simply for the fun of it is absolutely wrong."

3. Mark Aulisio and Robert Arnold, "Ethics Consultation: In the Service of Practice," *The Journal of Clinical Ethics* 14, no. 4 (Winter 2003): 279.

4. Both of which also differ from my use in chapter 3, in which I extend the con-cept to include broader social and ideological implications.

5. Christopher Meyers, "Cruel Choices: Autonomy and Critical Care Decision-Making," *Bioethics* 18, no. 2 (April 2004): 104–19.

6. Arthur Caplan, "Moral Experts and Moral Expertise: Do Either Exist?," in *Clinical Ethics: Theory and Practice*, ed. Barry Hoffmaster et al. (Clifton, NJ: Humana Press, 1989), 64.

7. Michael Bayles, "Moral Theory and Application," *Social Theory and Practice* 10, no. 1 (Spring 1984): 116.

8. A third version, casuistry, is also frequently cited as an alternative. I do not take it up here because its different versions give greater and lesser weight to the epis-temic priority of the initial, confidently held considered judgments that serve as the source for analogy to other cases. If they are held to be intuitively foundational, then those casuists are in some version of the "moral truth" camp assumed here. If, instead, the source of those judgments were something akin to a *volksgeist*, then my critique of the social consensus view, below, would apply to them as well. For fuller discus-sions see Albert R. Jonsen, "Casuistry as Methodology in Clinical Ethics," *Theoreti-cal Medicine* 12, no. 4 (December 1991): 295–307; Donald S. Klinefelter, "How Is Applied Philosophy to Be Applied?" *Journal of Social Philosophy* 21, no. 1 (Spring 1980): 16–26; and Mark Kuczewski, "Casuistry and Principlism: The Convergence of Method in Biomedical Ethics," *Theoretical Medicine and Bioethics* 19, no. 6 (Decem-ber 1998): 509–24. I also do not take up pragmatic approaches; for a powerful cri-tique, see Michael Bayles, "Moral Theory and Application," *Social Theory and Prac-tice* 10 (Spring 1984): 97–120.

9. Rosemary Tong, "The Epistemology and Ethics of Consensus: Uses and Mis-uses of 'Ethical' Expertise," *Journal of Medicine and Philosophy* 16, no. 4 (August 1991): 418. The third emphasis is added.

10. In addition to the already noted references in the *Core Competencies*, see also Mark P. Aulisio and Robert M. Arnold, "Ethics Consultation: In the Service of Prac-tice," *Journal of Clinical Ethics* 14, no. 4 (Winter 2003): 276–82; David J. Casarett, Frona Daskal, and John Lantos, "The Authority of the Clinical Ethicist," *Hastings Center Report* 28, no. 6 (November/December 1998): 6–11; and Nancy N. Dubler and Carol B. Liebman, eds., *Bioethics Mediation: A Guide to Shaping Shared Solutions* (New York: United Hospital Fund, 2004).

11. See Christopher Meyers, "Clinical Ethics Consulting and Conflicts of Interest: Structurally Intertwined," *Hastings Center Report* 37, no. 2 (March/April 2007): 2–10. I am grateful to Michelle Carter, John Hardwig, and Lisa Parker for their clarifying discussions of this point.

12. "Morality, Moral Theory, and Applied and Professional Ethics," *Professional Ethics* 1, nos. 1 & 2 (Spring–Summer 1992): 5–24 (emphasis added). I will take up this argument in greater detail below.

13. See Albert R. Jonsen, "Commentary: Scofield as Socrates," *Cambridge Quarterly of Healthcare Ethics* 2, no. 4 (1993): 434–38.

14. One argument is that medicine, being more scientific, has clear objective facts, while ethics is fundamentally about essentially and irresolvably contested concepts. Both premises are, I believe, mistaken; medicine is not an objective science and ethics is not hopeless relativism. For a nice discussion of this see Scott D. Yoder, "The Nature of Ethical Expertise," *Hastings Center Report* 28, no. 6 (November/December 1998): 12–13.

15. While versions of Jurgen Habermas's public discourse ethics are the predominant model and thus will be my focus here, see also Richard Norman's Wittgenstinian approach in "Applied Ethics: What Is Applied to What?" *Utilitas* 12, no. 2 (July 2000): 119–36.

16. Casarett et al., "The Authority," 7–8.

17. Quoted in Casarett et al., "The Authority," 8.

18. Distinctions could be drawn here among various kinds of relativism, ranging from the most narrow—personal subjectivism—to the broadest—something like "true for all humans," based on our contingent evolutionary history. If I read Habermas correctly, his is of the broader sort.

19. I am grateful to David Adams for his helpful suggestions here.

20. Casarett et al., "The Authority," 8.

21. For similar arguments see Iris Marion Young, "Communication and the Other: Beyond Deliberative Democracy" in her *Intersecting Voices: Dilemmas of Gender, Political Philosophy, and Policy* (Princeton, NJ: Princeton University Press, 1997), 60–74, especially 63; and Nancy Fraser, *Unruly Practices: Power, Discourse, and Gender in Contemporary Social Theory* (Minneapolis: University of Minnesota Press, 1989), especially ch. 8.

22. Sue Fisher and Alexandra Dundas Todd, *The Social Organization of Doctor-Patient Communication* (Washington, DC: Center For Applied Linguistics, 1983).

23. I am grateful to Roy Perrett for his many helpful suggestions in this section.

24. John Rawls, *A Theory of Justice* (Cambridge, MA: Belknap Press, 1971).

25. "Wide Reflective Equilibrium and Theory Acceptance in Ethics," *Journal of Philosophy* 76 (May 1979): 256–82, and "Wide Reflective Equilibrium in Practice," in *Philosophical Perspectives on Bioethics*, ed. L.W. Sumner and Joseph Boyle (Toronto: University of Toronto Press, 1996), 96–114. See also Yoder, "The Nature"; Jeroen Van Den Hoven, "Computer Ethics and Moral Methodology," *Metaphilosophy* 28, no. 3 (July 1997): 234–48; and Stephen Cohen, "General Principles and Specific Cases: Tension and Interrelation," *Professional Ethics* 6, nos. 3–4 (Fall–Winter 1998): 5–18.

26. Rawls, *Theory of Justice*, 19. It is important that these initial judgments not be given epistemic priority, else the position becomes some version of foundationalism. See Daniels, "Wide Reflective Equilibrium and Theory Acceptance," 265ff.

27. Rawls, *Theory of Justice*, 49f.

28. A common critique against traditional moral theory, especially Kant's, is that adherence to the theory forces moral judgments that are intuitively untenable. The value of coherence views, it is argued, is that the reverse can also work; that is, in determining the fit, confidently held judgments might force an adjustment to the theory.

29. Daniels, "Wide Reflective Equilibrium and Theory Acceptance," 268ff. See also Yoder, "The Nature," 13.

30. Yoder, "The Nature," 13, emphasis added.

31. Tom Beauchamp and James Childress adopt it in the later editions of *Principles of Biomedical Ethics* (New York: Oxford University Press, 2001). Cf., in the fifth edition, 397–401.

32. Daniels, "Wide Reflective Equilibrium in Practice."

33. Daniels, "Wide Reflective Equilibrium in Practice," 104–5.

34. Daniels, "Wide Reflective Equilibrium in Practice," 105, emphasis added.

35. While power asymmetries were no doubt not as striking as those found in most medical institutions, that difference would be one of degree, not of kind.

36. Daniels, "Wide Reflective Equilibrium in Practice," 110–12. I assume we must read the "surprise" as facetious (as is much of the playful-toned essay), since his theory assumes, even demands, such belief alteration.

37. I am grateful to Tom Campbell for his suggestions here.

38. Annette Baier, "Some Thoughts on How We Moral Philosophers Live Now," *Monist* 67, no. 4 (October 1984): 490–91, 492.

39. Sidney Callahan, "Ethical Expertise and Personal Character," *Hastings Center Report* 24, no. 3 (May–June 1994): 25.

40. Fear of such antidemocratic arrogance no doubt also underlies the Core Competencies' consensualist view.

41. Caplan, "Moral Experts," 73–74.

42. Caplan, "Moral Experts," 74.

43. Many hospitals are now considering a mandatory ethics consult for unilateral DNR orders. Others also "strongly recommend" a consult for cases involving perceived dual-patient conflict, for example, maternal-fetal conflict.

44. Some of the following recommendations are variants on those recommended by Yoder, "The Nature," 16–17, and Tong, "The Epistemology," 419.

45. The early trendsetter in this regard was the University of Tennessee Inter-Campus Graduate Program in Medical Ethics. Sadly, the clinical part of UT's program has in recent years been substantially reduced due to statewide cuts in higher education.

46. Tong, "The Epistemology," 419.

47. Patricia Werhane eloquently develops this idea in *Moral Imagination and Management Decision-making* (New York: Oxford, 1999). I will return to this key notion, along with additional arguments that reveal its richness, in chapter 4.

48. Aulisio and Arnold, "Ethics Consultation," 276–77.

49. Cf. Werhane, *Moral Imagination*.

50. See Meyers, "Clinical Ethics Consulting."

51. This interpretation was largely confirmed when the case manager succeeded in finding a long-removed legal relative. While the relative fully admitted to having been so long disconnected from the patient as to not really know him at all, she was nonetheless given decisional authority. Care was withdrawn and he peacefully died.

52. Aulisio and Arnold, "Ethics Consultation," 277, 279.

53. One of my early mentors was denied tenure when a dean who had promised that hospital work would justify a reduced number of publications retired. The new dean did not share these sentiments and it was too late to build a sufficient publication record. His case also reveals the importance of making sure that the tenurable value of such work activities is put into writing, preferably in departmental or campus tenure and promotion criteria.

# CHAPTER TWO

~

# Principles, Rules, and Character: A Model of Ethics Reasoning

To this point I have argued clinical ethicists should take a prescriptivist approach to clinical consulting. I now want to recommend a model that should guide their normative endeavors, one that is a variant on the principles-based approach so influentially recommended by Tom Beauchamp and James Childress.[1] I call it a "model of ethics reasoning" so as to avoid the extensive debate over whether this approach can rightly be called a moral theory.[2] Although I believe that discussion is in large part artificial (because it tries to draw an indefensibly sharp line between theory and practice), for my purposes little rides on the question; even if my recommended model is not theory, it is rooted therein, as should be clear in the arguments to follow.[3]

I admit from the outset that my recommendations are largely derivative, especially of Beauchamp and Childress's work. I see this part of the project as more of a synthesis, an attempt to take seriously and to flesh out Beauchamp's conclusion that their approach is not only consistent with, but closely allied with virtue theory and with theories that see the instructive elements of ethical reasoning as emerging from the often muddled details of case-driven moral decision-making.[4] That is, in this chapter I address four concerns related to a principles-based approach—their *source*, their *valency* through dilemmas, their *specificity*, and their *compatibility with virtue theory* (especially with respect to ethicists' educational role). I conclude, respectively, that little rests on resolving the source problem, that principles do retain valency in moral dilemmas even when outweighed, that principles' level of specificity is directly attached to the function they perform, and that a principle approach is not only compatible with virtue theory but may depend upon it.

## Principles

Principlism[5] begins with the notion that there are certain basic moral concepts that serve as normative guides. These guides, depending on their level of specificity, can serve either to motivate behavior directly or to justify and make sense out of other, more detailed, action directives. The modern progenitor of a principle-based theory, W. D. Ross, gave a "provisional" list of seven, referring to them as prima facie duties: fidelity (which is further divisible into promise-keeping and honesty), nonmaleficence, beneficence, justice, gratitude, self-improvement, and reparation.[6] Beauchamp and Childress narrow it to four, keeping nonmaleficence and beneficence (and thereby reinstating the distinction that William Frankena had conflated),[7] keeping justice (formal and distributive), and adding autonomy.

Although Beauchamp and Childress make a compelling case that nearly all moral considerations can be effectively subsumed under these four principles, I find in my teaching (both classroom and clinical) as well as in my own ethics reasoning that it is helpful to make some subdivisions. With Ross, I do not insist on the finality of this list. Rather, since it emerges from my review of others' work and from practical experience, more of either could well lead to amendment.[8] For now, the list looks like this:

- Respect for persons, that is, the Kantian notion that one should treat other persons, merely because they are moral persons, with great moral regard
- Nonmaleficence, that is, the Millian notion that one should avoid causing harm, whether physical, emotional, psychological, or economic
- Autonomy, that is, one should respect and promote others' autonomy, understood to be both, as per Kant, a structural capacity and, as per Mill, a disposition or an attitude of self-directed living[9]
- Trust, that is, one should avoid deception, both by commission and by omission[10]
- Reparation, that is, directly linked to nonmaleficence, when one does cause harm, one has a corresponding obligation to repair the associated damage
- Beneficence, that is, one should provide aid to those in need
- Merit, that is, one should receive appropriate reward for one's actions

- Distributive justice, that is, the Rawlsian notion that society's primary goods should be distributed in a way so as to reduce harmful inequalities.

Can these principles be hierarchically ranked? Strictly prima facie I would say so, and the list above represents my ordering. In the end, though, such a ranking does not have much relevance. Because the list *is* strictly prima facie and because I believe there is very little priority difference, even between respect for persons and distributive justice, circumstances will therefore almost always dictate which principle(s) should prevail in a given dilemma. The contingencies of specific cases produce their own hierarchies of duty.[11]

Also, I would argue, with Ross and Gert, that roles and relationships are directly relevant to the application of principles.[12] The prima facie strength of my obligation of beneficence is greater toward my child than toward someone unknown to me. In this and in all similar cases, though, the prima facie qualifier is again critical, as it is certainly not hard to imagine circumstances in which the obligatory stringency would be reversed. I will return to this point in the application section below.

## Their Source?

Given that so much of ethics reasoning rests on these principles, their source would seem vital. Answers have been many, including intuition, theology, naturalism, pure reason, utility, Aristotelian notions of practical wisdom, the consensualist and coherentist models described in chapter 1, and various contemporary versions of common morality and impartial reasoning.

In the early editions of their book Beauchamp and Childress make almost no attempt to justify their principles but instead more or less assume their validity and show how they can be used to make sense of the moral quandaries prevalent in health care. In later editions, after the sometimes harsh criticism noted above, they greatly expanded the justification section, moving toward a common morality and coherentist account. But even here a commonsense attitude seems to prevail, a sense of, "Oh come on, we should obviously respect and promote these principles. Hopefully theorists can work out their justifications, but for now we have real people facing real moral problems."[13]

This attitude can be traced to Ross's well-known, some would say infamous, claim that prima facie duties are self-evident; that is, they are intuitively known. As discussed in chapter 1, I find the coherentist model a powerful and potentially fruitful way to define and establish duty. I am also confident, though, that a coherentist process will produce a list very similar to the one described above. That is, my sympathies very much align with Ross; I realize this is not much of an argument (intuitive appeals, by definition, never are), but there does seem to be something about the nature of personhood that brings with it a recognition of the self-evidence of these basic principles.[14]

Ross does, however, leave considerable ambiguity over just how the prima facie duties are intuitively grasped. On the one hand he talks about them as "general principles that are recognized as self-evident," comparing them to the kind of knowledge persons have of mathematical propositions.[15] He also argues they are discerned through induction, that is, through experience of multiple cases that have inherent in them moral duty. When we encounter, for example, circumstances that include one or more parties having made a promise, we discern within those circumstances moral obligation. In our youth and immaturity we may not fully understand the nature of that obligation, but over time and with additional experience we learn to draw distinctions, to categorize the relevant duties.[16] As he puts it,

> There is nothing arbitrary about these prima facie duties. Each rests on a definite circumstance which cannot seriously be held to be without moral significance . . . [and] we see the prima facie rightness of an act which would be the fulfillment of a particular promise, and of another which would be the fulfillment of another promise, and when we have reached sufficient maturity to think in general terms, we apprehend prima facie rightness to belong to the nature of any fulfillment of promise.[17]

There is a kind of Aristotelian logic at work, a moving from the specific—particular acts with moral factors present therein—to the general—abstract moral duties applicable to a wide range of cases. Critically, though, abstract duties are not *learned*; rather, they are *recognized*. Again, they are self-evident and thus their validity is not *derived* from experience (as empiricists would claim). Instead, experience is necessary to produce enough cases for persons to achieve the "mental maturity" that provides, in a sense, *access* to the duties' self-evident truth.[18] Ross's theory thus represents an odd mix of necessary experience combined with direct knowledge. The experience does not produce the knowledge, but rather creates the conditions that make access to the knowledge possible.

A distinction is sometimes drawn here between such knowledge implying *truth* and such knowledge only implying *justification*. I do not think much rides on this distinction, or at least not for the type of analysis needed for my purposes. It may be such intuitions somehow provide direct access to genuine moral truth. It may be they can instead only be confirmed as part of some co-herently grounded system of beliefs. Or it may be they receive their epistemic priority through some as yet unexplained means. Any such answers would tell us *why* we should feel justified in making a knowledge claim, not *that* we should. While I hold out hope that metaphysical, epistemological, and, sub-sequently, moral theories will be developed that provide sufficient rational ground for accepting this type of knowledge as both justified and true, that ground is, I think, secondary to its practical value. And, as secondary, I see no particular problem even if the theoretical grounding never emerges. It is enough for me that principles very much like these have a seemingly unique phenomenology (i.e., our experience of them is direct and secure in ways most other beliefs are not) and that they are universally held. While there is very wide cultural disparity over their *employment*, some version of the prin-ciples is present in every known society.[19] It seems to be only skeptically minded philosophers who voice challenges, and such challenges, to my mind, usually come across as an intellectual *stance*, one quickly abandoned when faced with a true moral test.

An important qualifier, however, especially to the application of this method, is despite how Ross is sometimes read,[20] he is *not* an intuitionist when it comes to determining actual duty, or as he sometimes calls it, "duty *sans phrase*."[21] Actual duties are revealed only after extensive rational analy-sis. Intuition plays a role only when duties are in their prima facie state. Prima facie duties are self-evident, intuitively known, and general; for in-stance, persons should, all else being equal, keep their promises. Actual du-ties are those that emerge in specific circumstances, when one evaluates the competing duties at stake and determines which, in the case, should be acted upon. The first are known, Ross says, with certainty and are true for all per-sons; the second are closer to estimations. They are assuredly well considered, carefully and rationally reflected upon estimations, but they are nonetheless devoid of the intuitive certainty attached to duties in their prima facie state. The first are broad and abstract; the second are specific and contextual.

There is, admittedly, an odd metaphysics at work here, what I call "con-textualized absolutism." In their abstract, intuitively known state, principles are prima facie universal. This means four things. First, any rational, suffi-ciently mature person should recognize their prima facie normative force; that is, any such person should be able to independently come up with their own substantively similar list. Second, when the actual duty is correctly de-termined, it too is universal, that is, it holds for any person in relevantly like circumstances. Third, how principles are instantiated is wholly determined by context. The details of the dilemma—who and what are at stake—dictate which principles must be considered and in what manner. Another way of thinking of this is to say that, though universal, principles are not individually absolute. In the right circumstances, each may be overridden by other moral concerns, that is, by another, or multiple other, more binding principles. Fourth, the claim to epistemic priority applies only to the principles as abstract, not to a determination of actual duty. One cannot intuit which principle(s) should prevail in an ethical dilemma. In fact, the more complex the dilemma, the more principles at stake, the further one moves away from privileged, intuitive knowledge and the greater the possibility that one's ethical reasoning will be in error, due to mistaken facts or false conclusions about likely consequences.

This last point, about uncertainty, is in fact one of the more important aspects of this approach, in part because it reveals a sharp break from, especially, Kantian theories. Ross calls such uncertainty "moral risk" and says,

> Where a possible act is seen to have two characteristics, in virtue of one of which it is prima facie right, and in virtue of the other prima facie wrong, we are . . . well aware that we are not certain whether we ought or ought not to do it; that whether we do it or not we are taking a moral risk. We come in the long run, after consideration, to think one duty more pressing than the other, but we do not feel certain that it is so. . . . The judgement as to the rightness of a particular act is just like the judgement as to the beauty of a particular natural object or work of art. . . . Both in this [aesthetic case] and in the moral case, we have more or less probable opinions which are not logically justified conclusions from the general principles that are recognized as self-evident.[22]

Such uncertainty, though, hardly excuses an agent from engaging in careful moral reasoning. Indeed, on Ross's model, the reasoning is that for which persons can be held accountable. Again in Ross's terms, since we are not omniscient, since epistemic fallibility precludes our always being able to know "the good" (since we cannot with certainty know everything at stake in our choices nor what all outcomes will be), accountability is rightly attached only to doing "the right," that is, careful and sincere moral reasoning. If we do our best to determine the morally best choice but, through no reasonable fault of our own, get it wrong, we have done nothing blameworthy.

## Application

Hence, on this model, having a good method for moral reasoning is clearly vital. The first step in that process is a determination of the facts. Anyone who has done even limited ethics consulting knows that very often what appear to be value disagreements are instead factual ones. Clarifying what is really going on, getting everyone on the same page, often results in the problem simply going away. Such clarification generally requires good communication skills of the sort described in chapter 1. But, as I argue in chapter 4, the ethicist should also take an active searching and questioning role, rather than a passive, recipient one in which clinicians explain what is medically, and sometimes socially, at stake. They should because "the facts" will often include a much richer and subtler array of information than is typically presented in a standard case presentation, for example, institutional politics, underlying if unspoken normative rules, and participants' ideologies.

Even accepting this more active empirical role, however, the ethicist's primary expertise comes in determining what principles are at stake and in what ways. And again, after a careful and accurate review of the facts, ethicists will often determine only one principle is binding, or one principle is obviously far more binding, and thus the conflict is easily resolved: The facts are such and so; there is a clear, ethically principled reason to act; and relevant agents should thus respond accordingly.

The problem of course comes when, after the facts are made clear, multiple principles are at stake and they speak to different, even directly opposing, choices. How does one determine, in these cases, which principle or principles are most binding? How does one balance the competing principles?

## Balancing Principles

The approach defended here, first, holds that ethical dilemmas are real phenomena. A contrary view, rooted in theorists like Kant and Mill, argues that every moral problem has only one corresponding obligation, that is, the duty which is, respectively, consistent with the categorical imperative or with the promotion of the greater good.[23] Thus there can be no dilemma, no having to choose among competing obligations.

Because this conclusion appears so contrary to real persons' real moral experiences, many theorists either have tried to make the experience of conflict fit within standard theory or have moved away from such theory and toward a Rossian or other principlist account. As Barbara Herman puts it,

> One might hold that moral conflict is the stuff, the data, that moral theory ought to be about. If we started from experience instead of supposing that we have in place moral theory . . . we might take it that the determining data for theory is the experience of conflict and the need for its resolution. Our understanding of what moral principles are (or do) ought to accommodate that.[24]

It is just this that motivates Ross. In the following passage he uses the experience of conflict to reject both the Kantian line that promise-keeping is exceptionless and the consequentialist claim that the keeping of promises is morally relevant only insofar as doing so promotes the greater good:

> If I have promised to meet a friend at a particular time for some trivial purpose, I should certainly think myself justified in breaking my engagement if by doing so I could prevent a serious accident or bring relief to the victims of one. [Consequentialists] hold that my thinking is due to my thinking that I shall bring more good into existence by the one action than by the other. . . . However . . . it may be said that besides the duty of fulfilling promises I have and recognize a duty of relieving distress, and that when I think it right to do the latter at the cost of not doing the former, it is not because I think I shall produce more good thereby but because I think it is the duty which is in the circumstances more of a duty.[25]

Ross's argument here seems clearly right, both in its rejection of strict Kantian and consequentialist approaches and in its recognition that persons routinely experience, deeply *feel*, a conflict among prima facie obligations. To take a simple example, any reasonably informed parent has felt the moral conflict associated with giving a child an inoculation. The principle of beneficence creates a real and distinctly felt duty to provide the shot so as to protect against a devastating illness, while the principle of nonmaleficence creates a similarly real and distinctly felt—but competing—duty to protect the child from the inoculation's associated pain. In the vast majority of such cases, this is an easily resolved dilemma; that is, beneficence is, in Ross's language, "*more of a duty*" than is nonmaleficence.[26] Ross's important insight, though, is that it *is* a dilemma; two prima facie duties are present and both cannot be satisfied.

Most moral dilemmas are of course not so easily resolved, and thus a clear and effective method must be devised for balancing competing principles. Beauchamp and Childress and Gert take this requirement to heart and provide distinct but compatible methods. The following thus presents a melding of (some of) their conclusions.[27]

Assuming a sufficiently rich understanding of the relevant facts, including a determination of the principles at stake, a sound process of ethical reasoning requires the agent to undertake the following steps:

1. The agent must have and be willing to publicly state the reasons in support of her conclusion.
2. Those reasons must include an examination of harms (being avoided, prevented or caused) and of benefits (being promoted or lost).
3. The reasons cannot include nonrelevant considerations.[28]

4. The recommended actions must be consistent with the relevant and autonomous desires and beliefs of those beings most directly affected.
5. The intended goal must be realistically achievable (i.e., ought implies can).
6. There must be no less morally egregious option available and reasonable effort must be made to reduce or mitigate any concomitant harms.

While following these steps will, again, not produce infallible conclusions, done diligently, conscientiously, and sincerely, they help agents determine actual duty.

The potential for error gives impetus, however, to a seventh step—taking into account the valency of the overridden principles. Although not directly part of the determination of actual duty (and, hence, not discussed in that section by Beauchamp and Childress or Gert), the valency of principles is vital to full moral reasoning, particularly with respect to agents' moral engagement with the aftermath of decisions.

## Valency

The seventh step reads as follows:

7. In acting upon one or more principles, the agent must also keep before her the principles being overridden, not just so as to mitigate harms, but because she may now have a duty of reparation.

This "keeping before" is important because principles retain valency, continue to be morally relevant and to carry moral weight, even when overridden by other more binding principles. That is, in going through steps one through six, even when this produces the correct determination of actual duty, one does not therefore *negate*, or *undermine*, the other competing principles; rather, one only *overrides* them, or sees they are *outweighed* by those deemed more pressing. Those overridden still remain morally pressing; in contemporary language, they leave moral "residue."[29]

That principles retain valency is, admittedly, not a universally accepted view. The debate has emerged, in part, from the earlier noted question about the very possibility of moral dilemmas. If there are such dilemmas, the argument goes, this reveals there is moral value on either side (or the various sides) of the conflict. Thus when one side "wins," what happens to the other's value? Does it disappear or is there something remaining, something with moral force?

Beauchamp and Childress's limited references to the question of valency are decidedly ambivalent. They note, "It is misleading to say that we are, in these dilemmatic circumstances, obligated to perform both actions."[30] A couple of pages later, however, they say, "the agent who can determine which act is best to perform under the circumstances still might violate a moral obligation in doing so. Even the morally best action under circumstances of a dilemma can leave a trace of a moral violation."[31] This is striking not just because of the seeming contradiction—violating an obligation on behalf of another obviously entails that both obligations were initially present—but because of their choice of language. Many theorists prefer a weaker phrasing, that the "losing" duty is *overridden*, as opposed to being *violated*. This weaker terminology is often the preferred choice, I suspect, because of the discomfort associated with the suggestion that one can do right (acting on the more binding duty) while also doing wrong (violating a weaker duty).

Despite this discomfort, I think Beauchamp and Childress's second judgment is correct: The resolution of moral dilemmas necessarily involves violating one or more duties so as to promote those that are, in the case, more binding. The way to make sense of this rests in a careful consideration of both the kind of force attached to the concept of obligation and the ways in which prima facie duties create and sustain obligation.

## Force

One way of thinking about the kind of force attached to obligation is as implying a Kantian necessity, one that precludes the possibility of moral residue. Herman takes this route saying, "[B]eing obligated to do X implies that one may not omit doing X."[32] On this view it would be incoherent to conclude that in acting on one obligation others still remain, let alone that they are violated, since one cannot logically sustain two obligations, both of which are necessary and also mutually negating.

Herman does not, however, adequately explain why obligation must be understood as entailing necessity. She briefly addresses the point, but so far as I can see merely restates that which is under contention: "[I]f obligations do not necessitate, we do not generate the phenomenon of conflict of duty."[33] This simply seems wrong, both logically and with respect to how obligation language is routinely, and coherently, used. Different duties, even the same duty in different situations, carry varying degrees of moral force, all of which can engender conflict. Recall the earlier example of inoculating a child, where nonmaleficence was in conflict with beneficence. The moral force attached to the duty of nonmaleficence in this example is surely less binding than that present in the choice, say, whether to torture the same child in response to a sadist's offer to pay the child one hundred dollars while he watches you do so. Both involve conflict between nonmaleficence and beneficence, but with widely variable binding force. The torture case reveals a necessary obligation (one *must not* torture the child), while the inoculation case carries strong, but clearly overrideable force (one *should not* cause her pain from the shot).

This variability is also reflected in common usage of duties language, of both ordinary and scholarly types. Consider the range from the grateful ("much obliged"), to the morally relevant ("you ought to share your toy with your friend"), to the morally compelling ("you ought not lie"), to the morally necessary ("you must not cause gratuitous harm"). And, again, all these versions also can generate conflicting duties (e.g., gratitude can conflict with a claim of justice; the duty to share can be up against another to respect a parent's wish that the child not play with such toys; etc.).

Kant's distinction between perfect and imperfect duties is an acknowledgment of the differing degrees of force present in obligation, but even it seems far too limiting. Moral agents' real experience of facing and attempting to resolve a range of moral dilemmas reveals the force attached to obligation to be better understood as falling on a *continuum*, one capturing the full range of force pointed to in the above list.

At the opposite end from Herman are those who argue that prima facie duties carry *no* force. These theorists draw a hard and fast distinction between the respective degrees of obligatory force present in duties in their prima facie versus their actual states. On this view, prima facie duties are merely informative; they reveal what is morally at stake in dilemmas but they do not acquire obligatory force until made actual. David McNaughton describes them in this way:

> As he [Ross] points out, it is misleading to think of these as distinct or fundamental *duties*, since on his account prima facie duties are not strictly duties at all, "but something related in a special kind of way to duty." . . . The list might more accurately be thought of as a list of fundamental morally relevant characteristics of actions—of features of actions which are right- or wrong-making characteristics and which always carry weight when we are considering whether a particular action is right or wrong.[34]

Roy Perrett similarly characterizes them in his essay on a Buddhist, "middle way" approach to abortion. He says,

> To invoke the notion of prima facie duties in order to defend the permissibility of abortion is to give up the claim that there is a genuine dilemma of

abortion. Instead any apparent conflict of two moral obligations would be dissolved into a situation where only one of those obligations is actual. The other would then be merely prima facie (i.e. certainly overrideable, and perhaps not an obligation at all).[35]

Setting aside whether this is an accurate interpretation of Ross, there is still, I think, considerable room for valency on this reading.[36] That is, even if one grants that prima facie duties, as prima facie, are informative only, whereas actual duties carry moral force sufficient to guide correct action, reasoning over dilemmas also entails a third step, that of recognizing which duties are *at stake* in a given dilemma. This "being at stake" brings with it its own moral force.

The inoculation example again illustrates this point. As a reflective moral agent I recognize a range of prima facie duties—to be faithful, to show gratitude, to be just, and so forth. In this case I also recognize two of these duties to be both at stake and competing, that is, beneficence and nonmaleficence. They are at stake and carry moral force because, all else being equal, I am bound to do both—I am bound to protect my child from illness (beneficence) and I am bound not to cause her pain (nonmaleficence). Could I satisfy my latter duty without violating the former, I should surely do so. It is only because I cannot that I am justified in acting upon the *more* binding duty even though I thereby violate the *less* binding one. The qualifiers are emphasized because they reveal that both duties are present, at stake, with respective if unequal degrees of moral force. The less binding duty, though overridden, is not devoid of moral force; it just has less than the actual duty. And, contrary to Perrett's account, the lesser duty does not "dissolve"; rather, it remains cognitively present, morally relevant, even morally binding—that is, it has valency.

Perrett acknowledges this residue but, borrowing from Bernard Williams, sees it as an *emotional* reaction, present in the feelings of guilt, regret, remorse, and shame that exist even when persons genuinely believe they made the correct moral choice.[37] While I agree these emotions are often present, it seems inaccurate to reduce the considerations at work to these emotions, in large part because doing so restricts the experience of moral residue to a noncognitive *feeling* and because not having the feeling does not negate the valency; the agent could simply not recognize it. But just as the original prima facie duty has cognitive force, so also does the remnant. A more accurate account, I think, is that the emotions *reflect* the residue; that is, the emotion is not the residue itself but instead points to a genuine, cognitive awareness of duty. Morally aware and sensitive persons[38] *feel* guilt, regret, and the like precisely because they *cognitively recognize* the remnant obligation.[39]

These emotions can assuredly have *motivating* force, force often necessary to bolster an agent to act upon moral duty. This is of particular value when the moral residue includes a duty of reparation, a common remainder from dilemmas. One may realize that in doing the right thing, in acting upon one's best judgment of the actual duty, one has nonetheless committed a moral wrong, namely, violating the other competing and partially binding moral duty or duties. And thus, depending on just how binding were the competing duties, the extent to which one is accountable for the existence of the dilemma, and how efficacious any attempt might be, one may have a corresponding obligation to try to repair that wrong.

This way of thinking about how moral dilemmas are understood, addressed, and potentially resolved is admittedly messy and disconcerting, but it is also, it seems to me, far more reflective of real persons' actual decision-making. Morality is almost never about clear either-ors, strict right versus strict wrong. Instead, it is about embracing the complexity of mixed, competing, and overlapping duties and the associated obligations attached to resulting choices.

## A Process

From all this emerges a general picture of a principle-based process of ethical reasoning. An agent first determines what the factual issues are, including what principles are at stake. If a dilemma of conflicting duties is present, she analyzes it as per the steps described by Gert and Beauchamp and Childress. And she gives careful moral attention to any moral residue attached to the principles being violated, focusing especially on whether that residue creates a concomitant obligation of reparation.

A case will help illustrate the process. An eighty-four-year-old man was slowly dying from a wide array of problems: multiple strokes, kidney failure, inadequate lung function, deteriorating cardiac capacity, and an inability to eat on his own, all of which left him in a comatose state, fully dependent on life-sustaining (or, better, death-prolonging) technology. The patient was in the hospital's intensive care unit on a Medi-Cal reimbursement. He had no advance directive and his closest surrogate, his sister, insisted "everything be done to keep him alive." When pressed, she said, "God would provide a miracle," and proceeded to show the consultation team the letter she had received from a well-known national religious figure assuring her of the great likelihood of just such a miracle, if only she would continue to send regular donations "for prayer services," donations she was happy to provide.

The chair of the ethics committee, a cardiologist, had been called for a cardiac consult, the results of which motivated him to convene the ethics committee to determine whether continued treatment was futile. The committee evaluated the case as follows:

- Respect for persons. While members of the committee unanimously agreed such a prolonged death would be disrespectful to *our* conception of personhood, we had no evidence the patient felt similarly; indeed, the sister adamantly declared otherwise.
- Nonmaleficence. Because he was comatose, the patient experienced no pain. While one might argue his dignity and bodily integrity were being harmed, his sister again insisted he would have wanted all interventions, in anticipation of "the miracle."
- Autonomy. No other family member challenged the sister's status as the valid surrogate, thus we had to assume she was speaking as the patient would, were he able. Her reliance on religious authority certainly raised questions as to the extent to which her decision-making was truly autonomous, but no committee members were willing to deem her incompetent.
- Trust. All participants in the conversation were fully open and honest.
- Beneficence. If continued life was deemed a good, continued treatment was clearly beneficent.
- Distributive justice. This was the only principle that strongly supported withdrawal of care: Was this a just use of public resources, particularly at a time when California was going through yet another terrible budget crisis? As much as all the committee members wished otherwise, at least in this specific case, we agreed our public policy process left such determinations to state officials.[40]
- Reparation and Merit were not relevant to the case.

Thus we all agreed, with some distaste, the sister had the moral authority to insist on continued treatment. Further, we all felt comfortable with the reasoning process. That is, we examined harms, included only morally relevant considerations, clearly respected affected parties' autonomy, felt the intended goal (sustained life) was achievable, agreed there was no less egregious option available, and were willing to publicly defend our decisions.

We also all agreed, though, there were moral remainders, in particular concerns about whether the sister was being harmed by the seemingly unscrupulous religious authority, as well as continuing resource concerns. Thus the hospital chaplain (a member of the committee) agreed to continue to provide spiritual counsel to the sister. We also determined that should an ICU bed shortage arise—making this not just an allocation question, but one of triage—we would reconsider the case. As it turned out, to no one's particular surprise, the spiritual counseling had little effect beyond providing additional comfort and relief when the patient's body eventually just gave out.

Would a different outcome have resulted from a less systematic evaluation? I think so, as the committee chair came into the conversation convinced we could easily declare the treatment futile and use medical authority to override the sister's decisions. Only through careful analysis was he, and others initially sympathetic to his position, made to see that treatment was not futile (it clearly achieved the surrogate's intended goal—sustained life); that the sister's—and thus by extension the patient's—autonomous wishes carried strong moral weight; and that it was not our place to say this was an unjustified use of public resources. Again, the outcome was not one any of us would wish for ourselves or a loved one, but it was nonetheless ethically proper.

Two methodological concerns, however, remain. First, particularists argue that principles, even when they can be coherently explained and defined, remain hopelessly broad and vague, without sufficient specificity to be genuinely helpful action guides. Second, is principlism compatible with virtue theory? I take such compatibility to be of particular importance because I am convinced that a character approach is critical to effective ethics teaching and to motivating ethical behavior. I thus address each of these in turn in the remaining sections.

## Specificity

The problem of specificity lies at the heart of many of the most strident critiques against principlism: How can broad, abstract principles provide assistance with the day-to-day details of clinical life?[41] The criticism is also made against philosophers' reliance on abstract conceptual analysis. Combined, they are seen to result in a thoroughgoing rejection of principlism.

Although this book is also intended as a critique of the standard approach, I am, as preceding sections attest, still convinced of the vital role of theory and conceptual analysis in moral decision-making. The question, then, is whether it is possible to characterize and make use of principles in a way that they can provide real guidance in clinical ethics. They can, but only by recognizing that their meaning is variably specific or broad, as dictated by the context in which they are at stake. That is, just as obligation, force, and valency admit of context-dependent variability, so also does specificity.[42]

## The Problem

Jeffrey Blustein describes the problem as follows: "[E]ither principles are of limited specificity, in which case they are too coarse-grained to encompass all the particular features of detail and texture that give actions their moral significance to agents, or they are of unlimited specificity, in which case they cannot do any real justificatory work."[43] And the most frequent complaint is that philosopher-ethicists err far too often on the side of abstraction. Because of this, some urge replacing the conceptual/principle approach with a political or sociological model.

Barry Hoffmaster has become one of the more respected voices from the replacement camp. He says, "The principles standardly regarded as constituting the core of theoretical medical ethics . . . are too general and vague to apply determinately to concrete situations. . . . The real culprit . . . is a philosophical approach that creates and sustains the impression that moral theory and moral practice are discrete."[44]

He reaches this conclusion by way of three arguments. First, he says moral theory, like metaphysics and epistemology, is unrelated, in both development and structure, to real-world circumstances. Since it is not expected that other areas of philosophy will give us determinate truths or practical skills, "why, then, should moral philosophy be unique in having putative practical import?"[45] Second, the method of conceptual analysis can help clarify, but it will never rid medicine of "'essentially contested' concepts, like autonomy."[46] Third, "morality cannot be severed from the social, cultural and historical milieus in which . . . decision-making occurs."[47] Theory and principles, abstracted from context, cannot get at what is genuinely at stake and what clinicians are truly concerned with.

Many of Hoffmaster's conclusions accurately represent the reality of clinical ethics. Many consultants, trained in the standard approach, quickly realize they must adapt their method or risk being marginalized, at best only tolerated by clinicians. Too often, such ethicists' role is reduced to being little more than window-dressing for accreditation reviews. Clinicians, especially overworked residents and interns, care far less about, for example, the proper definition of autonomy than about whether someone higher in the pecking order will call them to task for not adequately respecting it, as that is institutionally understood. They are justifiably very impatient with overanalysis. As one intensive care unit director only half-jokingly put it, as he was excluding me from morning rounds, "I'll worry about *process* in M & M [mortality and morbidity] conference. Here, all I have time for is *outcomes*."[48]

Despite, though, how much Hoffmaster gets right, there is also much that is overstated. The meaning attached to concepts and principles does have to be context sensitive, but careful analysis, even in abstraction, can provide real guidance. When done well, it enhances understanding of the key background issues present in a range of concepts and principles, including autonomy, futility, beneficence, paternalism, justice, and informed consent. This can lead directly to changes in practice.

## Conceptual Variability

Take autonomy as an example. The concept is meaningfully expressed in general, abstract terms, for example, persons should be free to make choices consistent with their life plans. And this conception is wholly appropriate, for instance, for developing a broad institutional policy on informed consent that makes respect for individual choices near sacrosanct.

This same concept is also at stake, though, in a consultation regarding whether a patient with impaired cognition is sufficiently autonomous to be able to decide to withdraw life-sustaining treatment. For this question a much more nuanced application of the concept is required, one that takes into account, for example, the impact of illness and power asymmetry on voluntariness, on the level of informational detail necessary to make an adequately informed choice, on whether the agent has developed a habituated character trait of responsible decision-making (as opposed to routinely deferring to authority figures), and so forth.[49] Such situation-specific nuances reveal, contrary to the policy outcome attached to the abstract understanding, that on occasion a limited paternalism can actually increase a patient's autonomous decision-making by giving her the tools by which she can develop and act upon life goals. Again, the *same concept*, autonomy, is at stake in both circumstances and both applications accurately reflect its meaning and value.

## Practice Rules

This context-variable specificity can also be seen in how abstract principles get implemented through practice rules. As the principle is instantiated at increasingly specific levels, the principle-driven rule also becomes correspondingly specific. Take nonmaleficence. At its broadest, abstract level it captures the basic moral notion that it is wrong to cause harm, which then shows up at the societal level in a range of legal injunctions, such as the prohibition against battery. A bit more specific is the professional level, where, in the case of medicine, nonmaleficence appears in the well-known norm, "First and above all else, do no harm." Another level down is the array of hospital policies intended to protect patients from unwarranted harm (e.g., restraint regulations, staffing levels, conflict of interest rules). Finally, the principle gets expressed in the personal practice rules of individual physicians, such as where each draws the line regarding when the provision of pain-controlling morphine crosses the line into euthanasia.

In a like manner, a conceptual exploration of "futility" helps physicians see that even treatment that does not produce a cure can nonetheless achieve desired outcomes and thus by definition is not futile.[50] This in turn can have direct impact on patient care, as, for example, when one seeks temporarily to sustain terminal patients on life support so that families can arrive and say goodbye. Since, in my experience, most physicians rely on the cure-based definition of futility, they would be inclined to see such an action as pointless, giving them legal (and, in their minds, ethical) permission to dismiss the option outright. Through a careful analysis of the concept of futility, however, these same physicians can be made to see the range of problems with a cure-based definition, not the least of which is that it would make palliative care futile and thus also easily dismissed, since it does not achieve a cure. Working instead off a more sound definition—will the intended action achieve an agreed upon goal?—motivates a more thorough, and patient/family sympathetic, evaluation. That is, continuing to sustain the patient will clearly achieve the goal (helping to satisfy the family's emotional needs) and thus is not futile.

Granted, that goal must be subject to ethical evaluation, asking, for example, whether the family's needs ought to outweigh concerns over limited bed space. But that evaluation will be about issues other than futility. Similar conceptual arguments can be used to provide health professionals with a better understanding of power asymmetries (and how they affect informed consent), of what should count as unjustified medical harm, of the differences between and the relative strength of role-based versus personal obligation, and so forth.

### Not Either-Or

Each of these examples reveals just how valuable careful conceptual analysis is to ethical evaluation and to ethical practice. With it, one is better able to provide tools that help health care professionals make more informed judgments, better understand what moral issues and principles are at stake, and determine choices that reinforce patients' autonomy and enhance their and their families' well-being. Yet the temptation exists, it seems, to treat this methodological problem as an either-or: Either ethicists do abstract theory and conceptual analysis or they get down in the clinical muck and treat each problem as wholly particular with no uniform foundation to serve as a guiding rule. Daniel Chambliss seems to have bought into this false dichotomy:

The old [standard] model has become less and less realistic. . . . The logical der-
ivation of answers from principles (if it ever occurred) has certainly given way
to a mélange of standard operating procedures, stopgap measures, and tortuous
political compromises. . . . With the changes in medicine of the past twenty
years, [the standard model] has been reduced to an academic fantasy.[51]

Why, though, is being sufficiently attuned to clinical settings mutually ex-
clusive of theory? Good clinical ethics can, must, be both sensitive to the realities of institutional decision-making and informed by philosophically
grounded conceptual analysis. Recognizing the messiness of clinical contexts
need not push one into a foundationless relativism. By the same token, however, ethicists cannot treat real-world problems, and real-world people, as
mere abstractions.[52]

Thus, while critics like Hoffmaster are right that the standard approach is
not adequate, the adjustment must be one of *melding* the abstract with the
particular, not forgoing the former in the name of the latter. One key step in
such melding is to see the meaning of concepts and principles as being rich
enough to be understood as both broadly abstract and contextually nuanced.

I would also note that this same kind of conceptual analysis reveals that
these moral principles carry across professions and activities. Indeed, part of
a consulting ethicist's job is to remind practitioners in any setting that their
practice rules, if they are ethically sound, must ultimately be grounded in and
justified by abstract moral principles. For example, journalists often forget
that their practice rule of "getting the story," which they take to have normative content, must have a direct connection to the public's genuine right
to know, which is in turn justified by the principle of autonomy.[53]

Hence, in summary, the criticism that the principlist approach is too abstract and top down and thus can neither adequately appreciate nor effectively manage the gritty nuances of day-to-day clinical decision-making assumes principles are only broadly defined and applied. That assumption is
directly undercut when one recognizes just how rich in meaning the principles are, how they can be broadly abstract and narrowly specific depending
on the purpose for which they are being used, and how they get translated
into varying level-specific norms, policies, and practice rules.

And thus principlism emerges as a sophisticated tool for moral reasoning.
Principles have, according to context, variable specificity along with variable
obligation and moral force. They can be used to provide general guidance or
to determine best choices in concrete cases. And they can have compelling
force or they can be overridden in the face of other competing obligations.
Granted, this overarching variability makes the process of principle-based

decision-making tremendously complex; one cannot plug them into a formula and wait for the correct choice to emerge. The process requires instead a commitment to consider all the concerns present in these choices: For what purpose are the principles being used? What other principles are at stake? To what extent are the principles undercut by competing facts like illness and power? And so on. All these steps, though, are of course required for *any* sufficiently informed process of ethics decision-making.

With this understanding of principles in hand, what remains is accounting for the *person*, for the moral agent who will engage the principles. Humans, with all their quirks and character traits and flaws, still must employ the best method of reasoning. One standing criticism of principlism is that because it focuses on abstract principles whose existence is ultimately independent of persons, or at least of any given person, it therefore places insufficient emphasis on the *character* of moral agents. In the remaining section I show why this is an invalid criticism.

## Character

Once again, others have done the important groundwork on the connections between virtue theory and principlism. My goal here is to bring together and to elaborate on those arguments, particularly those of Beauchamp, Blustein, and Edmund Pellegrino.[54] Virtue theory's best contribution to principlism is found in its emphasis on discernment and motivation. In Beauchamp's terms, "[V]irtue theory is of the highest importance in a health-care context because a morally good person with the right motives is more likely to discern what should be done, to be motivated to do it, and to do it."[55]

Further, as Blustein notes, the process also works in the other direction—principles help create character:

> A person whose character is informed by a coherent set of principles has integrity in that he or she confronts the varying circumstances and predicaments of life with a certain constancy of moral outlook and purpose. Decisions on different occasions are not made solely on a case-by-case basis, but are guided and linked by a steady self-defining commitment to a certain way of living.[56]

When seen this way, the two theories emerge not only as compatible but as mutually complementary, even, in their respectively best applications, mutually dependent. They can only be taken as opposing theories, I think, if principles are held to be strictly external, not internalizable by moral agents. But such externalism is clearly false—principles can be, routinely are, internalized. They become part of agents' characters, part of their habitual way of thinking about and acting upon moral problems. They thus can enhance agents' characters and such characters, in turn, grant in agents the discernment and motivation to act in a principled way.[57]

### Educational Role

Most consulting ethicists also play an important educational role in the institution, and character development is at least as important there. The educational component of virtue theory is generally characterized through role modeling and experience, and the consulting ethicist has an essential part in each. In her own consultative activities she can become a role model, displaying various forms of integrity for emulation by students, residents, nurses, and even attending physicians. Such integrity can be expressed in a variety of ways, including compassion, open mindedness, careful diligence, reliability, honesty, benevolence, and fairness.

Indeed, as noted in chapter 1, these virtues are core elements of the humble attitude necessary for "expert" consulting. Also, given that the ethos of most medical institutions attaches expert status to the ethics consultant, she will and should be held to a higher standard. Outright hypocrisy is of course deadly to effective ethics consultation, but expectations here will likely be far more inclusive. Students and residents, especially, will want to see both a kind of technical expertise (i.e., the ability to give a complex and sophisticated analysis and potential resolution of difficult problems) and a genuine integrity, in order to believe they can rely upon the consultant for moral guidance. Such integrity is expressed in both obvious and subtle ways, for example, reliability, showing respect for all, offering assistance or a compassionate ear "off the clock," avoiding gossip and crass language, and declining residents' offers of "free" cafeteria food.

The consultant can also, in her teaching, point to other role models, especially others within the institution. Each institution has its version of the grand old matriarch/patriarch, persons whom all hold in high regard. Much of clinical education relies on case studies, and in these the ethicist can effectively include reference to the reflections and actions of such persons. Even better, if the person is available, the ethicist can occasionally bring her or him into educational sessions so the participants can directly observe her skills and character traits.

### Cases

Case study narratives also provide an indirect path to another component of character education, namely the experience upon which virtuous lives are

built, even if only experience by proxy. When cases are presented with sufficient vividness,[58] students can directly imagine themselves as participants in
dilemmas, learning from the described struggles, thought processes, successes,
and failures of the cases' decision-makers.[59] A more direct path, when possible, is to bring students into *real*, ethics-related case discussions. Doing so reinforces the ethical reasoning tools described above. It also provides a role
model to emulate and, of course, increases students' own experiences with
complex ethics decision-making.[60]

These are just some of the available methods for reinforcing character.[61]
The primary point, again, is that the virtues should be a central feature not
only in the ethicist's own decision-making, but in her educational role. Thus,
paraphrasing Beauchamp's conclusion, clinical ethics "is simply more complete if the virtues are integrated with principles."[62]

## Conclusion

Moral reasoning is thus a rich process involving careful analysis of facts and
theory, critical evaluation, complex skills, and developed character. Arthur
Caplan captures the mix when he says, "[W]hat is needed and what calls for
expertise, and perhaps experts, is the knowledge necessary to individuate,
identify and classify moral issues and problems in order to bring existing
moral perspectives . . . to bear."[63] That is to say, clinical ethicists must be able
to discern what *is* an ethical issue, evaluate its particularities as per the institutional setting, review the complex set of decision options, make a well-de-
fended recommendation, and provide appropriate role-modeling should it be
implemented. Caplan considers these skills the most important task of ethicists, more important than knowing and applying theory or principles.
Françoise Baylis echoes this sentiment, drawing upon the Aristotelian notion of practical wisdom or *phronésis* to describe the "practical 'know how'
whereby the focus of one's inquiry into a particular moral issue is on the different values and the ultimate aims of the various parties to the dilemma."[64]

While neither Caplan nor Baylis stresses the point, the arguments above
show that such practical wisdom must also rest within a virtuous character. Furthermore, as both Caplan and Baylis do emphasize, the ethicist cannot be a passive recipient of facts; rather, she must be sensitive to how the sources of information affect its nature, to the ways in which theory infiltrates facts, and to the
necessity for the ethicist sometimes actively to seek out additional information.

She must also, though, be cognizant of how clinical ethics cases are rooted
in and partly determined by a social context, one that reflects and reinforces
dominant social orders. Let me thus now turn to that argument.

# Notes

1. Tom Beauchamp and James Childress, *Principles of Biomedical Ethics*, 5th ed. (New York: Oxford University Press, 2001).

2. See Bernard Gert, "Moral Theory and Applied Ethics," *Monist* 67, no. 4 (October 1984): 532–48. See also the series of articles in the *Journal of Medicine and Philosophy*: Bernard Gert and K. Danner Clouser, "A Critique of Principlism" 15, no. 2 (April 1990): 219–36, and from the same issue, Ronald M. Green, "Method in Bioethics: A Troubled Assessment," 179–97. See also, B. Andrew Lustig's reply, "The Method of 'Principlism': A Critique of the Critique" 17, no. 5 (October 1992): 487–510, and Green, Gert, and Clouser's reply to Lustig, "The Method of Public Morality versus the Method of Principlism" 18, no. 5 (October 1993): 477–89.

3. For more of the debate on the relationship between theory and practice in principlism, see the series of essays on principlism in Raanan Gillon and Ann Lloyd, eds., *Principles of Health Care Ethics* (New York: John Wiley & Sons, 1994), especially the essay by Gillon, "The Four Principles Revisited: A Reappraisal," 319–33. See also three articles in the *Hastings Center Report* 31, no. 4 (July–August 2001) by Onora O'Neill, "Practical Principles and Practical Judgment," 15–23; Martin Benjamin, "Between Subway and Spaceship: Practical Ethics at the Outset of the 21st Century," 24–31; and Margaret Olivia Little, "On Knowing 'Why': Particularism and Moral Theory," 32–40.

4. Tom Beauchamp, "Principlism and Its Alleged Competitors," *Kennedy Institute of Ethics Journal* 5, no. 3 (September 1995): 181–98.

5. Gert and Clouser were the first to use this term, and they meant it to be derogatory, Gert and Clouser, "A Critique." Beauchamp and Childress and their supporters, though, seem to have unreservedly adopted it as a shorthand description for their approach, and thus I do so here as well.

6. W. D. Ross, *The Right and the Good* (Oxford: Oxford University Press, 1930), 19–24. Ross called them "duties," and because I think nothing more than style rests on the different terminology, I will use the terms interchangeably in what follows.

7. William Frankena, *Ethics*, 2d ed. (Englewood Cliffs, NJ: Prentice Hall, 1973).

8. In addition to the sources cited in notes 1–4 and 6, see Stephen Cohen, "General Principles and Specific Cases: Tension and Interrelation," *Professional Ethics* 6, nos. 3–4 (Fall/Winter 1998): 5–18, and the bibliography compiled by Pat Milmoe McCarrick, "Principles and Theory in Bioethics," *Kennedy Institute of Ethics Journal* 5, no. 3 (September 1995): 279–86.

9. Christopher Meyers, "Cruel Choices: Autonomy and Critical Care Decision-Making," *Bioethics* 18, no. 2 (April 2004): 104–19.

10. Worded this way, it seems to me, trust captures the wide range of associated concerns, including promise keeping, fidelity, and honesty. It might be, however, that these should each be identified as separate principles.

11. For an interesting interpretation of Ross on this problem see David McNaughton, "An Unconnected Heap of Duties?" *Philosophical Quarterly* 46, no. 195 (October 1996): 433–47.

12. Ross, *The Right and the Good*, 19, 22, 38; Bernard Gert, *Morality: Its Nature and Justification* (New York: Oxford University Press, 1998), 211–12.

13. Beauchamp gives a more extensive defense of these foundations, in response to yet additional criticism, in "A Defense of the Common Morality," *Kennedy Institute of Ethics Journal* 13, no. 3 (September 2003): 259–74. In this essay he distinguishes between the common, and *universal*, morality and what he calls "particular moralities," that is, those rooted in subcultural or professional norms. I fully agree that different contexts bring different morally relevant *facts* (see chapter 4), but I think, with Ross, were one to correctly interpret those facts, one would come up with the absolutely correct answer. Hence my characterization of this approach as "contextualized absolutism" (see below).

14. For a fuller account of this point, and of what follows, see my "Appreciating W. D. Ross: On Duties and Consequences," *Journal of Mass Media Ethics* 18, no. 2 (2003): 1–18.

15. Ross, *The Right and the Good*, 31, and 30, 32–33.

16. As, again, he says we do with mathematics, where sufficient experience is necessary to move from concrete examples to a recognition of abstract necessary truth.

17. Ross, *The Right and the Good*, 20, 33.

18. Ross, *The Right and the Good*, 29.

19. The Ik are commonly cited as an exception to this empirical claim. While there is some debate as to whether the Ik abandoned all morality (i.e., whether they retained a principle against gratuitous harm), even if they did, one would be hard pressed to call the circumstances of dire extremis they faced sufficient to retain any semblance of "society." See Colin Turnbull, *The Mountain People* (New York: Touchstone Books, 1987).

20. Cf. Alan Donagan, "Moral Dilemmas, Genuine and Spurious: A Comparative Anatomy," in *Moral Dilemmas and Moral Theory*, ed. H. E. Mason (New York: Oxford University Press, 1996), 18–19. See McNaughton, "An Unconnected Heap," for an interpretation closer to mine.

21. Ross, *The Right and the Good*, 18.

22. Ross, *The Right and the Good*, 30–31. See also 31–32, in which he discusses the relationship between "good fortune" and the right act. Beauchamp and Childress echo this lack of certainty: "We cannot hold persons to a higher standard in practice than to make judgments conscientiously in light of the relevant norms and the available and relevant evidence," *Principles*, 22.

23. I borrow from Beauchamp and Childress in my definition of a moral dilemma as a situation either in which good reasons support, but do not conclusively support, both sides of competing obligations, or in which competing positive duties are present, but in acting on one, the other is necessarily overridden, *Principles*, 10.

24. Barbara Herman, "Obligation and Performance: A Kantian Account of Moral Conflict," in *Identity, Character, and Morality: Essays in Moral Psychology*, ed. Owen Flanagan and Amélie Oksenberg Rorty (Cambridge, MA: Bradford MIT Press, 1990), 314. As the title suggests, Herman attempts in this paper to show how Kant's theory can accommodate moral dilemmas. I will take up part of her argument below.

25. Ross, *The Right and the Good*, 18.

26. For illustrative purposes I intentionally make the example simple, setting aside any potentially serious harms associated with the vaccine itself (e.g., actually giving the child the disease).

27. Beauchamp and Childress, *Principles*, 19–20, and Gert, *Morality*, 17–18. The melding here is admittedly artificial since Gert does not so much describe a balancing of principles (in his language "rules") as discuss the circumstances in which they may be violated. The approaches are, I think, sufficiently similar as to make it a sympathetic melding, a conclusion Beauchamp also reaches, "Principlism," especially 186–90.

28. Beauchamp and Childress say, "The agent must act impartially in regard to all affected parties; that is, the agent's decision must not be influenced by morally irrelevant information." If they include as morally relevant one's special role-based obligations, as Gert (and Ross and I) would, then their language here is compatible with Gert's public impartiality requirement combined with his sixth, "position" clause.

29. See Terrance C. McConnell, "Moral Residue and Dilemmas," in Mason, ed., *Moral Dilemmas*, 36–47.

30. Beauchamp and Childress, *Principles*, 10.

31. Beauchamp and Childress, *Principles*, 12.

32. Herman, "Obligation and Performance," 312.

33. Herman, "Obligation and Performance," 315. This tactic is understandable given that her primary argument involves a reconsideration of the "ought implies can" dictum as a way of retaining a Kantian necessity in obligation while also acknowledging a conflict in duties.

34. McNaughton, "An Unconnected Heap," 435.

35. Roy Perrett, "Buddhism, Abortion, and the Middle Way," *Asian Philosophy* 10, no. 2 (July 2000): 110. Perrett's interpretation is consistent with that given by Jonathan Dancy, "An Ethic of Prima Facie Duties," in *A Companion to Ethics*, ed. Peter Singer (Cambridge, MA: Blackwell Books, 1991), 219–29.

36. It should be clear that I interpret Ross to be assigning moral force to prima facie duties, even if it is to a lesser degree than that existing in actual duties. In fact, much of the argument to follow emerges from my attempt to make sense out of Ross's difficult and confusing discussion of parti- and toti-resultant attributes, Ross, *The Right and the Good*, 28–33.

37. Perrett, "Buddhism," 106–7.

38. Jeffrey Blustein plausibly argues that the kind of moral sensitivity required here is rooted in moral virtue and character, a point I will take up below: "Character Principlism and the Particularity Objection," *Metaphilosophy* 28, nos. 1–2 (April 1997): 135–55.

39. Perrett has since agreed that this analysis of duties is both compatible with his paper's primary argument and possibly a better way of thinking about prima facie duties. Personal communication, November 2001.

40. Most committee members also agreed this is wise public policy; health care professionals should not be resource gatekeepers at the bedside of their patients.

41. Cf. Jonathan Dancy, "Ethical Particularism and Morally Relevant Properties," *Mind* 92 (October 1983): 530–47; Stephen Toulmin, "The Tyranny of Principles," *Hastings Center Report* 11 (December 1981): 31–39; Barry Hoffmaster, "Can Ethnography Save the Life of Medical Ethics?" *Social Science and Medicine* 35, no. 12 (1992), 1421–31; and the influential book by Stephen Toulmin and Albert Jonsen, *The Abuse of Casuistry* (Berkeley: University of California Press, 1988).

42. For related arguments see Beauchamp, "Principlism," 190–93; Beauchamp and Childress, *Principles*, 15–18; and Blustein, "Character Principlism."

43. Blustein, "Character Principlism," 140.

44. Hoffmaster, "Can Ethnography," 1422.

45. Hoffmaster, "Can Ethnography," 1421–22. Many epistemologists, I suspect, would challenge his claim that their work cannot give "practical skills," especially those doing research in such areas as studying whether testimony provides justified belief. Cf. Robert Audi, "The Place of Testimony in the Fabric of Knowledge and Justification," *American Philosophical Quarterly* 34, no. 4 (October 1997): 405–22.

46. Hoffmaster, "Can Ethnography," 1422–23.

47. Hoffmaster, "Can Ethnography," 1428.

48. As noted in the introduction, this mentality has also given rise, in the corporate world, to the emergence of in-house "ethics officers," the vast majority of whom are not philosophers but are results-oriented practitioners who come from within company ranks and receive varying levels of ethics training at workshops and conferences. The *Economist* reports that such "ethics officers, who barely existed a decade ago, have become *de rigueur*, at least for big companies. The Ethics Officer Association, which began with a dozen members in 1992, has 650 today." April 22, 2000, 66.

49. Meyers, "Cruel Choices."

50. While there is still debate over the correct definition of "futile treatment," the best discussions are those that meld careful philosophical analysis with clinical realities. See for example Howard Brody's argument, which is to my mind convincing, in "Bringing Clarity to the Futility Debate: Don't Use the Wrong Cases," *Cambridge Quarterly of Healthcare Ethics* 7, no. 3 (Summer 1998): 268–72.

51. Daniel Chambliss, "Is Bioethics Irrelevant?" *Contemporary Sociology* 22, no. 5 (September 1993): 649–50. See also Arthur W. Frank, "First-Person Microethics: Deriving Principles from Below," *Hastings Center Report* 28, no. 4 (July–August 1998): 37–42.

52. Carl Schneider provides an excellent, reality-based critique of an abstract model of autonomy that treats all patients as "hyperrational," independent agents, all seeking and all capable of fully autonomous informed consent. See *The Practice of Autonomy: Patients, Doctors, and Medical Decisions* (New York: Oxford University Press, 1998).

53. See my "Justifying Journalistic Harms: Right to Know vs. Interest in Knowing," *Journal of Mass Media Ethics* 8, no. 3 (Summer 1993): 133–46.

54. Beauchamp, "Principlism," especially 193–95; Blustein, "Character Principlism"; and Edmund Pellegrino, "Toward a Virtue-Based Normative Ethics for the

Health Professions," *Kennedy Institute of Ethics Journal* 5, no. 3 (September 1995): 253–77. See also the insightful discussion of the relationship between principles or rules and virtue theory in chapter 1 of Rosalind Hursthouse's *On Virtue Ethics* (New York: Oxford University Press, 1999).

55. Beauchamp, "Principlism," 195.

56. Blustein, "Character Principlism," 148.

57. Blustein also points out how a character approach helps explain moral residue, in that a person of character "will also experience moral distress in response to the recognition that she has deceived others even when, all things considered, this was the right thing to do." Blustein, "Character Principlism," 147–48.

58. Martha Nussbaum's work on storytelling and moral imagination eloquently captures this point. See, for example, *Love's Knowledge: Essays on Philosophy and Literature* (New York: Oxford Press, 1992), and *The Fragility of Goodness: Luck and Ethics in Greek Tragedy and Philosophy* (Cambridge: Cambridge University Press, 2001).

59. Role models can of course be *negative* as well as positive, and negative ones are often more powerful motivators. (I am grateful to Keith Horton for reminding me of this.) Using institutionally connected persons as negative role models, though, is much more politically risky and thus one is probably better suited by pulling such examples from a distance.

60. The emphasis on direct experience is central to casuistry, the version of particularism most often taken to be especially compatible with virtue theory. For fuller discussions see Toulmin and Jonsen, *The Abuse*; Albert Jonsen, "Casuistry as Methodology in Clinical Ethics," *Theoretical Medicine* 12, no. 4 (December 1991): 295–307; John D. Arras, "Getting Down to Cases: The Revival of Casuistry in Bioethics," *Journal of Medicine and Philosophy* 16 (February 1991): 29–51; and Mark Kuczewski, "Casuistry and Principlism: The Convergence of Method in Biomedical Ethics," *Theoretical Medicine and Bioethics* 19, no. 6 (December 1998): 509–24.

61. See also Edmund Pellegrino and David Thomasma, *A Philosophical Basis of Medical Practice* (New York: Oxford University Press, 1981).

62. Beauchamp, "Principlism," 195.

63. Arthur Caplan, "Moral Experts and Moral Expertise: Do Either Exist?" in *Clinical Ethics: Theory and Practice*, ed. Barry Hoffmaster, Benjamin Freedman, and Gwen Fraser (Clifton, NJ: Humana Press, 1989), 81.

64. Françoise Baylis, "Persons with Moral Expertise and Moral Experts: Wherein Likes the Difference," in *Clinical Ethics*, ed. Hoffmaster et al., 96.

# CHAPTER THREE

~

# Social Context and the Politicization of Clinical Ethics

"There is a deep sense in which clinical ethics consultation is more in the domain of the political than the moral and more in the domain of practice than theory."[1]

Clinical ethics cases occur within a social context. Their causes, their potential solutions, their very identification *as* ethics cases are in large part determined by the context in which they are embedded. Context serves as the foundation for clinical ethics, and yet the clinical ethics literature gives it scant attention, emphasizing instead a case-study methodology that generally assumes independently autonomous decision makers.

That absence is particularly striking given that much of the more widely construed bioethics literature,[2] especially early work and that focusing on the economics of health care,[3] has been directly concerned with macrolevel structural analyses. Many such theorists conclude, in fact, that these analyses are requisite to bioethics. For example, Howard Waitzkin argues:

Major problems in medicine are also problems of society; the health system is so intimately tied to the broader society that attempts to study one without the other are misleading. . . . These interconnections are not only important for clearer understanding; they also suggest directions of change. From this view, health reforms that do not address the relationships between the health system and broader social structure are doomed to failure.[4]

Also, importantly, macrolevel bioethics work has often had an at least secondary agenda of recommending rearrangements of political and institutional structures so as to make them more consistent with general ethical principles, in particular with principles of justice. In part because of this agenda, such discussions have also played an important role in informing debate, particularly as issues like informed consent and patients' rights to refuse treatment have worked their way through the courts. That influence is also present in current debates on health care reform and genetic engineering.

Yet, again, little of such socially grounded analysis has found its way into the reams of material written on the clinical ethicist's proper role. That literature mainly treats ethical issues as if they exist in a social void, unaffected by social, cultural, or institutional beliefs, attitudes, and norms.[5] Cases are presented as standing in isolation, involving little more than the specific medical facts and the relevant principles or values, and solutions are seen as individual, not structural or even institutional. Discussions often include questions about legal options and, sometimes, concern about impact on the family's financial resources, but there is almost never the kind of structural analysis that so informs the best macrolevel work. And, as Waitzkin rightly avers, "too narrow an analysis not only overlooks the dynamics that create and reinforce specific problems but also obscures directions of meaningful reform."[6]

Part of the reason for the absence of structural analysis is revealed in the following comment from an anonymous journal reviewer's reaction to an earlier version of this argument. In response to my claim, detailed below, that clinical ethicists must expand their skills base and scope of analysis, she or he writes: "Many clinical ethicists would hold that the relevant expertise of the ethicist is knowledge of ethical concepts, theories, and traditions. . . . Why expect the ethicist rather than the social worker, psychiatrist, or advertising psychologist to provide" the relevant parts of a multifaceted structural analysis? This attitude is also echoed by Aulisio and Arnold: "Emphasizing 'ethics' at the expense of facilitation and mediation . . . runs the risk of portraying ethics consultation as primarily an intellectual exercise in ethics."[7]

As I argued in chapter 2, ethics need not, should not, be conceived of so narrowly as these quotations would suggest. Again, ethics is not just about understanding and applying abstract concepts, principles, and theories. It is assuredly about those things, but it is also about understanding how those abstractions reside within a social framework, how psychology and institutional politics motivate ethical conflicts, and how effective communication and mediation are critical to finding solutions to such conflicts.

And it is about the structural norms that underlie cultural communities; that is, it is about social context, or so I want to argue in this chapter. I will, first, give a brief explanation of the nature of social contexts; second, show how typical case commentaries reveal and reflect such context; and, third, discuss how the work of clinical ethicists would differ were they to adopt a structural approach. I conclude by arguing that at least some clinical ethicists, in some circumstances, should advocate change of those social, political, and institutional structures that regularly produce the kinds of dilemmas arising in clinical settings.

This chapter also represents an extension of the prescriptivist argument from chapter 1, in that I continue to urge ethicists to advocate the morally preferable alternative, but now with the added claim that this should be done through a politically informed lens. That is, using the vernacular common to political movements, I conclude ethicists should also be *activists*.

## The Nature of Social Contexts

Social contexts are complex entities that incorporate ideology, power, the law, cultural norms, religious beliefs, professional values, and institutional cultures. So as to focus the discussion here, I will speak mainly of the broad rules and guidelines that motivate and guide members' behavior. These structures are analogous to how grammar functions in language, dictating both how to participate in a practice in a meaningful way and what counts as normal, acceptable behavior.[8]

For example, a partial list of the structures currently present in U.S. health care includes a rejection of any form of single-payer plan, especially socialized medicine; a class-based variability in standards of care; an acknowledgment of the status and power of physicians, present culture-wide, but particularly so in direct clinical encounters; an at least superficial appeal to patient autonomy;[9] a faith that new technologies will solve old and emerging medical problems; a rejection of death as natural and even sometimes a blessing;[10] a continued gendering of illness, particularly of mental illness (e.g., depression and anxiety), with different medical responses to and treatment options for men's and women's respective ailments; a belief that certain illnesses, for example, alcoholism, drug addiction, sexually transmitted diseases, and smoking-related pulmonary diseases, are the result of patients' voluntary choices and are thus less deserving of empathetic care; and an acceptance that diseases engendered by environmental pollutants are a natural part of modern life, for which medical response, rather than social overhaul, must be developed.

This list is not intended to be exhaustive, in part because what one includes is no doubt largely determined by one's ideological orientation. The specific content of the list, though, is much less important than a recognition that there is one, that deep structural factors directly influence the provision of health care and thus also influence ethical issues therein.

The notion of a social context, and of its concomitant political and institutional structures, is rooted in an extensive literature of Marxist, phenomenological, and political thought. A full explication would require considerably more detail than is appropriate here, but two key components are important. First, social context theory holds that persons make sense out of their world in part by viewing it through political, normative, and ideological frameworks or schemas.[11] Such schemas determine what agents consider normal, natural, "common sense,"and thus also what is *noticed*.[12] In Alfred Schutz's language,

> the existence of the [schema] and the typicality of its contents are accepted as unquestionably given until further notice. . . . All problems arise on the background of what had been given as unquestionable . . . and all solutions of problems consist in transforming, by the very process of questioning, that which has become questionable into something new.[13]

For example, accepting that humans are carnivorous is a powerful structure in the United States. As such, appeals to a vegetarian diet are *noticed*, sometimes even seen as a form of propaganda. By contrast, meat-based diets are seen as the norm, taken for granted.[14] Similarly, physician-patient power asymmetries are so grounded in how persons approach health care, they go *unperceived*; they are part of our culture's understanding of contemporary medicine. Awareness of them occurs only when something unusual occurs, when a physician badly abuses her power or when a patient attempts to reverse or even balance the symmetry.

Second, social context is in the main transparent to its members; it is part of the given, of that which is taken for granted. Members within a social context generally do not recognize it *as* one, since its values, beliefs, and norms simply *are*, which also helps explain its general absence from the clinical ethics literature. In the midst of clinical work, the typical clinician—or clinical ethicist—does not give explicit attention to, for example, the structural rejection of single-payer compensation schemes, nor does she consider how that structure may be contributing to the problems present in the case at hand. The focus is instead on the immediate details of the case. Later, over a cup of coffee or a beer, she may bemoan the economic state of contemporary health care provision, but only in the manner of philosophical reflection; such musings generally play no role in her treatment plans or actions because she does not see the structure as directly present in, even a direct cause of, the case's relevant facts.

Depending, though, on how well defined and powerful are the context's structures, they can often be made explicit by outsiders, including by clinical ethicists. This puts such ethicists in a potentially powerful position—immersed enough in the clinical environment to have a thorough understanding of its structures, but also enough of an outsider to critically evaluate them. My argument is thus that the clinical ethicist should shift her focus to include those structures and their impact upon clinical ethics problems.[15] Doing this represents a significant shift in clinical ethicists' focus and purview, but doing so will alter how she analyzes problems as well as her resulting recommendations.

## Cases in Context

"In approaching a physician for help, a patient brings not only a physical problem but also a social context," writes Waitzkin.[16] And yet, "the patients and doctors in these encounters seem to accept the social context as given; . . . *criticism* of the social context remains absent."[17] For such criticism to occur, social structures must be made apparent.

One way to do this is to look at examples of case-study reviews, and there is no better source for these than the *Hastings Center Report*. A multiyear review reveals that commentators focus on narrow clinical and legal concerns; structural evaluations are almost wholly absent.[18]

I obviously cannot provide an analysis of every published case. Instead, I have taken three cases, from three different decades, chosen because they discuss predominant clinical ethics issues. And while I believe them to be paradigmatic of these kinds of case reviews, I don't try to prove that here, since one could suggest that the cases were picked precisely because they confirm the hypothesis. Instead, my goal is to show what a structurally informed case analysis looks like. My hope is the reader will then be able to discern how different this approach is from the standard version and can directly compare it to other published case reviews.

I repeat the cases in full and as originally written, summarize the commentators' responses, and show how a politicized version would differ. I want to stress that the kinds of analyses provided by the commentators are, on the whole, insightful, helpful, and important; they are just too narrow.

## Advance Directives

The first case is "Whether 'No' Means 'No,'" with commentary by Lewis Silverman and Manette Dennis and by Fenella Rouse and David Smith.[19]

Dr. D is an emergency physician in a large urban hospital. One relatively quiet evening Mr. R, a thirty-two-year-old male, presents to the emergency department complaining of shortness of breath. The problem, as it develops, is a depressingly familiar one to Dr. D. Mr. R, known to be HIV positive, turns out to be having his first episode of pneumocystis pneumonia, an often fatal disease of AIDS patients. The episode, fortunately, appears at present to be a relatively mild one; his blood test shows his lung function is only moderately impaired.

When Dr. D begins to explain this, Mr. R insists that his friend Mr. U be brought into the emergency department to listen to the doctor. Dr. D goes over the condition and describes the appropriate treatment: IV antibiotics. When asked, Mr. R denies any drug allergies.

As they grapple with the news that Mr. R has now changed from being a patient with HIV to one with AIDS, Mr. R and Mr. U produce a living will and durable health care proxy form designating Mr. U as responsible for decision-making if Mr. R becomes incompetent. The living will forbids cardiopulmonary resuscitation and prohibits under any circumstances endotracheal intubation and respirator ventilation, along with various other measures. Dr. D believes strongly in patient autonomy. He therefore assures Mr. R and Mr. U that Mr. R's wishes, as clearly expressed, will be respected. After arranging for the papers to be copied and placed in the chart, he goes to admit Mr. R and Mr. U leaves.

While a bed is being readied, Dr. D orders a dose of the appropriate antibiotic to be given to Mr. R and goes to see the next patient. Upon starting the antibiotic and leaving the room for a few minutes, the nurse returns to find Mr. R unresponsive, with a bright red rash and severe trouble breathing. Immediately recognizing a life-threatening allergic reaction, she stops the antibiotic and calls for the doctor.

Mr. R is in anaphylactic shock. Quickly ordering the four appropriate medications, Dr. D opens his mouth to ask for an endotracheal tube and respirator and realizes he has a problem.

Mr. R will die as his airway closes up if patency is not immediately ensured by placement of a tube. Indeed, in a case like this, placement often requires cutting the patient's throat to maintain the rapidly narrowing airway. Seconds, quite literally, count. The good news is that this is a time-limited condition. With immediate aggressive action, only a few hours or days of ventilator support should be necessary and there should be absolutely no long-term sequelae. Of course, it is possible that Mr. R's pneumonia will acutely worsen. He might then be unable to be weaned off the respirator. An emergency physician with no experience in the long-term management of either pneumocystis pneumonia or anaphylaxis, he is unsure of the chances of that.

What should Dr. D do?

The microlevel clinical issues are relatively straightforward. As both commentaries note, Dr. D missed an important opportunity to clarify what was truly meant by the categorical prohibition against intubation, since it is the unusual patient who in fact means "under any circumstances." And, as Silverman and Dennis indicate, intubation could easily be reversed, should the surrogate determine this situation in fact falls under an intended blanket refusal.

A deeper analysis, though, reveals political structures vital to a thorough case review. First, why must Mr. R "insist" that Mr. U be included in the discussion? If this were a heterosexual couple, especially one believed to be married, the default would be reversed, that is, unless the patient insisted otherwise, the spouse would have been at the bedside all along. While there could be reasons other than structural bias against gay couples behind the initial exclusion (e.g., concern about disruption of the treatment), it is nonetheless telling that the commentators do not note the issue, since the exclusion is strongly suggestive of how antigay attitudes influence clinical cases.

There are also two structural considerations present in the poor communication. Dr. D is portrayed as a physician who does not use his position of power to reject the couple's expression of control, yet his total acquiescence to their fairly irrational request reflects how structural communication problems, rooted in power, still exist in medicine. The commentators imply that Dr. D's failed communication is unusual; in my experience, it is the norm. That is, as the power asymmetry between physicians and patients gradually lessens, physicians have yet to learn how to have a healthy, power-*balanced* relationship with patients. Many well-meaning physicians, having embraced the value of patient autonomy, treat control as either-or; either they have near total control of the medical encounter, or the patient does. Cases like this one, though, demand a true balance, one in which the physician sufficiently realizes the appropriateness of questioning a problematic, even irrational, advance directive and at the same time respects the patient's autonomous authority to choose her own health care. Such balance is difficult in any human relationship, and historical power structures make it especially hard in health care.

A last, related structural problem is also one of the more pervasive in clinical care and thus one of the more important for ethical analyses. If better communication were to occur, Dr. D would have to try to get at why Mr. R is so adamantly opposed to aggressive treatment. While probably no one wishes to die under the full court press of a contemporary critical care unit, the rational alternative is not *no* aggressive treatment. Part of Mr. R's motivation, if we are to take him to be typical of patients in similar circumstances, is a fear of a prolonged, painful, and medically torturous death. That he sees this as the *only* alternative to no treatment is irrational; that he sees it as the *likely* alternative to no treatment is fully rational, which speaks directly to endemic problems present in U.S., hospital-based, end-of-life care. Rouse and Smith touch on this concern, but they treat his reaction as misguided, easily fixed by a better conversation with Dr. D. They do not acknowledge the structural problems in U.S. hospital care that engender a *justified* fear of aggressive treatment.

## Surrogate Consent

A variant on this problem is present in the second case, "Proxy Consent for a Medical Gamble," written by Dennis Saver, with commentary by Ronald Carson, Henry Aranow Jr., and Nancy Rhoden.[20]

Norma Walker left her job when six months pregnant. Nine days after the baby was born she experienced severe headache, fever, and a mild reaction to light. The next day, Sunday, she met with her obstetrician in the hospital emergency room. He found no abnormalities and felt strongly that further evaluation by an internist was imperative.

Since Ms. Walker did not know an internist, she and her husband were worried about finding a physician who would come to the emergency room on a Sunday morning. Dr. Stanley, a physician whom they both knew personally, happened to be in the emergency room at the time, and Mr. Walker asked him to assume care of his wife. Her obstetrician agreed.

Dr. Stanley learned that the Walkers' two-year-old child had recently had viral meningitis, as had several other children and adults living near their home. When reached by phone, their pediatrician confirmed that two children had been proven by lumbar puncture to have aseptic meningitis and had been treated conservatively at home. During the interview the Walkers expressed anger about the impersonal and unpleasant way Ms. Walker had been treated by hospital personnel in the labor and delivery suite a week earlier. Mr. Walker was especially bitter and was certain she would have had better care at home.

The results of laboratory tests showed that Ms. Walker probably had a just-beginning viral meningitis (for which no specific treatment is necessary), but may have had a bacterial meningitis (a life-threatening illness requiring treatment with intravenous antibiotics).

The test findings were carefully explained to the Walkers. Dr. Stanley stated that because of the circumstances, the chances of Ms. Walker having viral meningitis were very high. But the result of the spinal fluid test raised the possibility of bacterial meningitis. The physician argued that, if he or his wife were the patient, he would play it safe and go into the hospital for two days of intravenous antibiotics until the spinal fluid culture was complete.

Ms. Walker felt too ill to think clearly—she would, she said, do whatever her husband decided. Mr. Walker was determined to be involved in the decision. He was clearly concerned for his wife, but wasn't sure whether "playing it safe" was the best course of action. He appreciated the personal favor of the physician who agreed to undertake her care on short notice and had given a detailed explanation of the medical evaluation. However, her recent hospitalization had left a bad impression. Also the couple had no insurance. Was the small chance really much of a gamble? Mr. Walker needed time to think and went for a walk.

Upon returning, he announced his decision—to take the gamble. He would take his wife home, fully aware of the risks and of Dr. Stanley's discomfort with his decision.

Who ought to have made the decision about treatment in this case? Was Mr. Walker's decision justifiable?

All three of the commentators treat Mr. Walker's decision as problematic, with reactions running the gamut. Rhoden suggests that if the medical facts are as ambiguous as the case suggests, the physician has to treat the husband's choice as "far from ideal [but] justifiable." Carson concludes Dr. Stanley should "insist" upon hospitalization, implying that physician authority would likely be sufficient to change Mr. Walker's mind. And in the unlikely case the Walkers still choose to depart, at least "the physician will not have encouraged that decision by offering them a choice which is not theirs to make." Aranow is even more adamant. He calls Mr. Walker's decision "appalling" and says that "to permit the mother of two children, who has a central responsibility to their care and upbringing, to run such a risk because of her anger and that of her husband 'about the impersonal and unpleasant way she had been treated by hospital personnel in the labor and delivery suite a week earlier' strikes me as, in the highest degree, unwise and irresponsible."

Three structural problems are present in the case. The first again raises the question of the harsh treatment too often experienced during hospitalizations. The Walkers are presented as generally reasonable, loving people who care for each other and their family. Thus their unwillingness to face another hospital stay, even with the potential threat to Ms. Walker's life, has to be treated as powerfully motivated; reasonable people do not choose such potential risk without feeling impelled to do so. Carson acknowledges that "hospital care is often brusque and inconsiderate, at times even unkind. Patients understandably recoil from such treatment and seek to avoid it." But he then goes on to conclude that Dr. Stanley should attempt to browbeat the Walkers into acquiescing to be treated the same way again. None of the commentators speaks to reassuring the Walkers that such treatment is unacceptable and that steps will be taken to ensure that they would not face such problems with this hospitalization. The unspoken attitude is instead, "Yes, patients are treated very badly in the hospital and this is a shame, but we just have to live with it." But patients should not have to live with it; rather, the attitude expresses an ideology of power: Patients, especially poor patients with limited health care options, simply have to put up with what the medical establishment imposes upon them and when they object, their choices are deemed "appalling."

Second, the commentators give almost no consideration to the Walkers' concerns regarding insurance. In fact, the only mention of it is in Rhoden's backhanded compliment that the husband's economic concerns did not suggest his "motives were suspect." A two-day hospitalization, the case implies, represents a serious strain on their resources, particularly if they had to hire someone for child care. This reality gives the "gamble" very different odds. It is one thing for persons of relative wealth to say it is not worth the risk; it is something altogether different for those for whom two days in the hospital would represent a serious burden.

Third, and maybe most disturbing, is the pervasive sexism in the case. None of the commentators make note that Ms. Walker so easily hands the decision off to her husband. Up to that point she is presented as being sufficiently coherent and competent to engage in a complex conversation. Yet, at the time of decision, she allows her husband to determine, potentially, her very life or death. It is not necessarily that Dr. Stanley should have challenged the power dynamics present in the couple's relationship; it is that the commentators do not deem those dynamics worthy of mention. Far worse, though, is Aranow's explicitly sexist comment, "to permit the mother of two children, who has a central responsibility to their care and upbringing." If the characters' roles had been reversed, it is hard to imagine Aranow chastising the husband in the same manner, worrying about *his* "central responsibility."

This case is the oldest of the three (1980), and while such blatant sexism likely would not show up in a similar case commentary now, I still regularly hear comparable comments in the clinic. And the case paradigmatically reveals the presence of political structures, of power asymmetry between medicine and patients, of disregard for the difficulties of the poor, and of blatant sexism. None of this is acknowledged in the commentators' evaluations. In fact, Carson claims to the contrary when he says, "The decision required in this case is a medical one," implying that by being so, it is therefore also divorced from social context.

## Resisting Treatment

The third case is "Resolution and Ambivalence," with commentary by Miriam Cotler and by Linda Ganzini and Lewis M. Cohen.[21]

Ms. B is an eighty-six-year-old widow who lives in a California retirement home. She is a gentle, sociable lady and likes to reminisce about her work doing make-up for movies. She has no family locally but does have one good friend nearby and a 101-year-old sister on the East Coast. She is in the hospital for treatment of an infection, from which she is recovering. She also has chronic kidney failure, however, and has been on dialysis for about eighteen months.

For at least the past eight months, Ms. B has told her doctors, her nurses, and her friend that she wants to stop the dialysis. She understands that her life depends on receiving it, but she hates the process and does not want to live this way. Yet she continues to board the van that takes her to the dialysis center three times each week. She claims that every time she tells her doctor she wants to stop, he describes the risks of falls, fractures, and a miserable end.

Even with the dialysis, Ms. B has been hospitalized three times after falls or for pneumonia. In fact, the current hospitalization occurred after a fall in the dialysis center. Each time she is ill, her statements about discontinuing are stronger, although when her nephrologist comes by on his rounds, she is quiet and appears to accede to treatment. With others, however, her cries to stop the treatment are ever more persistent, emphatic, and emotional. She complains that this is not what she wants, that her doctor frightens her and makes her feel guilty, and that some of the nurses encourage her to hold onto and to try to enjoy life. She says that her wishes are clear and her instructions ignored, but she also admits that she is confused about whether it is truly right to exercise her will to discontinue the treatments.

> A consulting psychiatrist concludes that she is oriented, competent, and severely depressed, as evidenced by her wish to discontinue treatment. He prescribes Prozac. But how should we read the case? What ought to be done about Ms. B?

The commentaries show a greater appreciation for political structures, but still come up short. Ms. B's situation screams of power asymmetry; for example, she pushes hard to have her autonomous wishes respected except when dealing with the nephrologist, the person on her treatment team who, as the specialist, holds the greatest institutional power. In his presence she "accedes" to his wishes; that is, she allows his authoritative voice to override her own.

If Ganzini and Cohen notice this, they certainly downplay it. The only hint of it is in their comment that physician support for a dialysis patient's decision to stop treatment has been found "to be the essential factor" in whether that decision is respected. But instead of pursuing this to discuss the need to reduce such physician power, they conclude "physicians must learn to actively listen to patients' requests."

Cotler does better, recalling Jay Katz's and Howard Brody's exhortations to notice power asymmetries in physician-patient relationships. But this point comes relatively late in her commentary, only after wondering whether there might be factors in Ms. B's history—"prior relationships, habit, heritage, the influence of family, and other personal and social factors"—that that would account for her "irresolution." That question also suggests Ms. B's case is unusual, that a possible "lifetime of pleasing and deferring to" more assertive persons explains her difficulties with the nephrologist. But one need not appeal to a speculative history to make sense of her acquiescence. The facts of the case explicitly point to a well-established medical phenomenon—patients, even those of relatively strong will, routinely accede to physician authority.[22] Cotler's approach, in fact, comes across as a variant on blaming the victim. It is not Ms. B's personal history that is to blame, but an endemic structural power asymmetry.

Cotler does nicely pull out a second structural problem in the case, that of, as she puts it, "Prozac to the rescue." The evidence of Ms. B's "severe depression" is not so much that she wants to discontinue dialysis, but that she does so in the face of authority figures' recommendations to the contrary. If the roles were reversed, that is, if the nephrologist felt it was time to let go and she wanted to continue treatment, you can be sure the psychiatrist would not be prescribing *him* Prozac! Cotler, however, disappointingly does not point out the other obvious structure here, that of genderized treatment. If it was Mr. B, the odds of his being diagnosed as severely depressed and in need of Prozac are slim. Ganzini and Cohen's commentary leaves out all mention of the problems associated with the psychiatric response.

## Differing Recommendations

Again, I have no quarrel with the commentators' microlevel recommendations, at least in the first two cases. I also do not want to devalue that level of ethical engagement; it is necessary to a full review. Such a review extends to include the political and institutional structures embedded in, and partly determining of, the related medical encounters and concomitant ethical problems.[23]

One might argue that in the limited space typically available for these kinds of published case reviews there is not enough room to address both the micro- and macrolevel concerns. My recommended shift in focus, however, does not require substantially more words; rather, it calls for a different way of looking at cases, with differing responses naturally following, as described below. If it is not realistically possible to provide both micro and macro analyses in a limited case review, why should the micro hold priority? Determining priority cannot be an a priori process, but rather can emerge only out of the specific considerations in each case; sometimes the micro should take precedence, sometimes the macro. Furthermore, the focus of my argument is to motivate changes in clinical ethics consulting, that is, within the clinical environment, where space/time limitations are not quite so restrictive. I rely here on published reviews because they are the only reasonably available source for analysis and because such reviews, appearing as they do in the field's leading journal, naturally guide practicing clinical ethicists.

How, then, should an inclusion of the political affect what an ethicist does and recommends in actual cases? That is, what sorts of changes, particularly in outcomes, should it produce? In response to the first case, if the ethicist brought a structural approach to her work, she would educate staff about the inclusion of obvious partners—married or not, heterosexual or not—in appropriate patient conferences. She would also emphasize, in her hospital teaching, the importance of power-balanced relationships and communication. And she would work both to change standard critical care so that it is not so tortuous and to give patients more power and greater control over treatment options.

Those latter activities would also clearly be appropriate in response to the second case. Additionally, the ethicist should work to sensitize practitioners, especially relatively well-off physicians, to the genuine health care–related hardships faced by the poor. Sometimes this is as simple as pressing that point in rounds; sometimes it requires activism at the social level. Finally, while an ethicist probably cannot change deep-seated bigotry (sexism, racism, etc.), she can work to make sure such biases do not impact patient care discussions, in part by making the biases explicit when they occur.

The differences would be even more direct in the third case. Recognizing that the patient's autonomous decision-making was being compromised by the physician's authoritative voice should result in an immediate intervention. The patient essentially needs an ally, someone who can balance the nephrologist's power in their clinical conversations. The ethicist could handle this herself or she could recruit another physician, one who better understands and respects the patient's wishes. Such an ally would serve either to convince the nephrologist to abide by Ms. B's choices or to give her the power to reject his position. The ethicist could also use the case as an opportunity to discuss with the psychiatrist the pervasive gender differences in mental health treatments.

All of this points to a broadening of the clinical ethicist's scope. It also brings some degree of personal risk, that is, in job security. How politically involved, then, should clinical ethicists be? This question is a natural continuation of the argument so far. Having extended what should be included in case analyses, and having realized in doing this the impact of political structures on clinical encounters, the ethicist is left with a dilemma: How far should she go in trying to alter or replace those structures that consistently have a negative impact? I already concluded, in chapter 1, that well-trained and competent ethicists have a unique expertise, one that justifies their taking a more prescriptive clinical role. Does that same training and competency qualify one for activist structural reform? It is one thing to recognize the impact of political and institutional structures on medical encounters and to include this realization in one's clinical ethics analyses and recommendations; it is another to take an activist position, to push to alter or replace such structures.

## Activism

A personal anecdote will help motivate this section. One of my graduate school clinical ethics internships included an eight-week stint at a state mental health facility. As the weeks progressed, it became clear the kinds of issues the hospital administration, and to a lesser extent our faculty, expected us to explore were of a relatively superficial sort; that is, they did not touch on the underlying institutional and social structures that motivated the problems in the first place. Thus for my culminating project I picked one of those structural problems and, working with some of the hospital staff, developed a plan for real reform.

During the exit interview, the hospital administrator devoted the entire hour to a discussion of the appropriate role of ethics consultants—and especially ethics students—arguing, in the end, that such activism was outside our appropriate purview. His view was, as argued above, certainly consistent with that held by most others in our field.

In this section I argue not only that it is *appropriate* for philosopher-ethicists to be ethical activists but that they *should* be, that they do a disservice to their role otherwise. In making this case I address three related questions: first, whether there is an obligation to promote change; second, whether philosopher-ethicists are relevantly qualified and can be effective; and third, whether decisions within practical settings will benefit from this push for structural reform.

### A Duty to Be Activist?

On the obligation question, I align myself with the many beneficence-centered arguments that conclude that human beings have a clear obligation, within reasonable limits and individual competencies, to improve the situation of others and to work to reconceive institutions that produce harm. This general claim is well established in utilitarian and other beneficence theories and the relevant arguments need not be repeated here.

Is there, though, a specific, role-related obligation of clinical ethicists to actively promote beneficial outcomes, that is, to take an activist stance? Should moral or political activism toward institutional structures be part of the job description of clinical ethicists? Jorge J. E. Garcia thinks not: "Keep philosophers out of [public life], for they do not have what it takes. . . . Our job seems to be rather to criticize and to challenge . . . but we should not compromise our nature. This means that we have a role in public life, but it is an indirect role, as teachers and critics, not as advisors and active participants."[24]

Garcia is not clear on the point, but the "nature" he does not want compromised seems to mean the kind of objectivity often taken to be the professional standard for the classroom, that is, that philosophers should carefully and fairly represent all sides of an issue without advocating any. The classroom environment, though, is enough different from clinical consulting, even if one concludes that an attempt at such classroom objectivity should be the norm,[25] it does not follow that the same standard should apply here.

Furthermore, Garcia sidesteps that philosopher-ethicists have a historically grounded obligation of professional service, service attached to their status as members of a privileged profession. While nearly all universities now interpret that to mean service to one's campus (predominantly through committee work), the requirement historically also had a community focus. Part of the academy's very purpose was to provide *public* service, both out of a recognized duty of beneficence and in appreciation for the social status and prestige afforded its members.[26] To claim, as Garcia does, we fulfill this service requirement indirectly, through teaching, mentoring, and committee work, ignores that these are activities for which we are directly compensated.

A second reason our role demands activism is connected to the recognition that all reform-minded activists risk personal loss; their activities, by definition, challenge existing power. For academically rooted ethicists, however, this threat is substantially lower than that faced by others similarly well positioned to effect change. Many clinical ethicists are employed primarily in academic departments and either have or are on the road to tenure. Clinical ethics for these persons is thus a side job.[27] And the culture of their primary workplace—academia—tolerates, even encourages, political analysis, activity, and dissent, all within the security of guaranteed employment.

Third, some medical-center physicians also have tenure with an affiliated academic institution, but most are too enmeshed in the professional and institutional ethos to be truly effective critics.[28] And those institutional employees not so culturally enmeshed are also, maybe even by definition, persons without much institutional power and thus vulnerable to political backlash. While they might otherwise be well positioned to be potent critics, any such activity could well represent a direct threat to their job security. Compare this to the typical philosopher-ethicist whose job is secure and who has legally grounded and culturally reinforced academic freedom.

This does not mean there is *no* threat to the clinical ethicist. These are often great jobs, providing unique job satisfaction and, frequently, considerable monetary compensation. But many hospitals still see an ethics consultant as a nice but hardly necessary member of the staff. Thus, if the clinical ethicist is perceived as creating problems through political activism, some administrators and powerful physicians might use this as an excuse to cancel the position. Much of this, however, is mitigated by differing expectations attached to the outsider's role (a consideration I will return to in a moment). And, in any case, the potential sacrifice for the typical clinical ethicist is significantly lower than for other institutional employees, assuming she has a tenured position to fall back upon.

From this emerges my first conclusion of this section: Clinical ethicists' uniquely privileged position brings a special duty to try to effect change. In short, if many are aware of the need for change and some can act accordingly with limited personal risk, surely those persons have a greater obligation to do so.

## Efficiency

A second reason has to do with outcomes. Namely, there is a kind of efficiency in being activist.[29] As revealed above, political structures like gender bias, classism, and professionally based power asymmetry in medical encounters are often the root causes of specific case conflicts, even if they are not explicitly present to the participants. Thus, if the ethicist does nothing to bring about structural change, related ethical problems will appear and reappear. Such change can be either formal (i.e., changing relevant laws or institutional policies) or informal (i.e., changing institutional practice).

Take as an example the structural bias, present in the first case above, toward legal marriage and against nonlegal partnerships, a bias that is also frequently antigay. California, like most states, has case law–based requirements that legally recognized relationships take legal precedence over nonsanctioned partnerships. This structural bias regularly produces absurd outcomes, like physicians struggling to obtain consent from physically and emotionally far-removed legal next-of-kin (or, worse, the never formally divorced ex-spouse) while a ten-year partner sits in the waiting room. Many persons in nontraditional relationships try to get around bias by assigning durable power of attorney for health care to their partner, but they still often encounter strong resistance from bigoted clinicians. Furthermore, it is still only a fraction of the general population who holds such advance directives.

A range of activist responses is available to the ethicist here. At the formal level she can advocate changes in state law that would grant legal status to gay, lesbian, and straight partnerships, or she can advocate a formal change in hospital consent policy. At the informal level she can educate staff to rely, in practice, on partners' consent. For example, medical residents can be taught that proxy consent is best obtained from the person or persons closest to the patient and thus most familiar with life goals and values. Then, as necessary, they can request legal next-of-kin to legally sanctify the already agreed-upon treatment options.

While this approach has the value of practical efficacy, it probably skirts around the letter of the law.[30] Furthermore, even though physician authority is usually sufficient to acquire such formal sanctification, it is not always so, especially when, as is typical, the process occurs by phone. The far-removed next-of-kin, knowing her legal rights, often insists on taking control, even sometimes traveling cross-country to be present at the bedside. Sometimes this is done out of genuine beneficence and concern, sometimes it is done out of denial, sometimes it is an intentional rejection of the new partner, some-times it is rooted in unresolved family issues. In the clear majority of such cases, though, the outcome is worse, given time delays, given the need to get the new consenter caught up on relevant medical, ethical, and economic is-sues, given frequent family conflicts, and given the new consenter's reduced knowledge of the patient's goals and values.

In short, the informal approach, while often helpful, does not get at the root problem—a legally sanctioned structural prejudice. If the ethicist wishes to reduce the occurrence of these all-too-common problems, she has to be an activist, pushing to alter the legal, social, and institutional structures that generate the conflict.

## Problems

Ought, though, of course implies can. To say consulting ethicists have the obligation entails they have the ability, the *competence*, to fulfill it. And as Garcia makes clear, it is not at all obvious ethicists have, in his words, "what it takes" to do this right.

This concern takes us back to my arguments in chapter 1 regarding the requisite knowledge, skills, and temperament to be an effective ethicist. These also overlap with those necessary for activism. The ethicist/activist needs appropriate training in how to analyze problems—getting at their nor-mative underpinnings so as to evaluate the moral stakes and thus ultimately to be able to give good advice. She also needs the right temperament, that is, she needs to care deeply about producing better ethical processes and out-comes and she needs the humility to realize her own failings.

Furthermore, the ethicist/activist needs to be well situated to analyze in-stitutional structures. She needs to be immersed in the medical environment without being enmeshed in its culture. Sound structural criticism requires deep familiarity with the relevant issues, people, and frameworks. Yet at the same time critics must retain a sufficient distance so as not to become incul-cated in the ethos. This is obviously a fine balancing act—being sufficiently aware of the ethos while not being subject to it—but one clearly manageable by the conscientious person, particularly when she is only a part-time con-sultant with external, and secure, employment.[31]

The outsider status also allows ethicists to "get away with" critical evalu-ation of political and institutional structures in a manner insiders cannot. Power players often do not feel as threatened when criticism comes from out-siders. There is not, normally, residue from former battles, concern over turf, political maneuvering, and the like. Often the outsider is given credence just because she *is* an outsider, someone who can bring a perspective relatively free of institutionally based biases.

Retaining one's position as a critical activist outsider also helps the clinical ethicist avoid one of the core problems attached to the role—being co-opted. The problem, in a nutshell, is determining to whom the ethicist is beholden. Robert Veatch voices the concern as follows:

> Clinical ethicists . . . ought to be making themselves available primarily to the primary decision makers. . . . If choices are to be made by patients, then clinical ethicists ought to have the patient as the primary client. The fact that the ethicist is on the clinician's turf, is paid by the health professional system, and gradually develops identification with clinical professionals, all cast doubt on the legitimacy of the clinical ethicist's role.[32]

Gerald Dopplet puts it similarly. The ethicist, he says,

> who functions effectively as a consultant, gaining credibility and authority among physicians, over time and as a matter of institutional habit, undoubtedly internalizes their routines, and utilizes them much of the time as his touchstone of what is reasonable and ethical. She becomes an "in-house ethicist" and leaves the wider, more reflective standards of philosophy (applied ethics) behind.[33]

Medicine is a seductive environment. The status, the money, the trappings of power, the *actual* power all contribute to a context in which it is easy for a consulting ethicist to be co-opted. The key consideration is one of self-definition and thereby of *attitude*. If the clinical ethicist defines herself as a member of the institution, she will internalize its values. But if she sees herself as, at least in part, a structural critic, if she retains a politically informed approach to her work, she is more likely to keep considerations of justice at the forefront and will better resist being co-opted. If she conceives her role in large part to be activist, to strive to change the very systems that would likely tempt, she is less likely to be seduced by them.

I learned this lesson, and the subtle processes of internalization, from someone in a position normally that of the consummate insider—the then-director of the intensive care unit where I do most of my consulting work. I was asked to assist on a case in which the family expressed deep distrust of the physician team and of the institution. While a healthy skepticism toward physician advice is not unwarranted, in this particular case their distrust was resulting in a loved one being sustained on life support far beyond what was otherwise consistent with his and their values; that is, they all agreed he should not be kept alive if all it meant was delaying death, particularly if it meant pain for him and wasteful use of resources, all of which, unfortunately, were the case. They just did not *believe* it to be the case. My job was to facilitate more effective communication between the family and the treating team, so the family could better trust what they were being told, thereby helping them to act upon their explicitly stated goal of allowing their loved one to die when appropriate. In the midst of the conversation I, unthinkingly and without awareness at the time, said "we" when referring to the hospital's position. While it evidently had no impact upon their eventual choice (they decided to withdraw all treatment and he died in relative ease), the ICU director very rightly later pointed out the error of that language. By its use I communicated to the family that I was not a neutral advisor but was in fact on the hospital's "side."

Also, again harkening back to the argument from chapter 1, a prescriptive role can actually work against co-option, in main part because it gives power to the ethicist. In addition to the seductive quality of the medical environment, the other main contributor to co-option is a sense that one is subservient to, and serves at the whim of, more powerful persons. In this environment, one cannot help but tend toward the obsequious, always striving to be taken seriously, to be treated with respect, to be in good with the "big dogs." Thus a role that serves to legitimate, and give power to, the consulting ethicist by structurally assigning her an activist, challenging function will dampen the co-option threat.

Still, though, ethicists may have good skills at recognizing the nature of problems and the need for change but still be weak at knowing how to achieve it. For example, most clinical ethicists sorely lack key political skills: What will be the political ramifications attached to a particular recommended change? Whose power will be threatened and how can they be appeased? How can coalitions be built that can achieve change even in the face of strong opposition? And how will such changes affect institutional resources or outside funding? Such skills are not normally within most clinical ethicists' training. They can be acquired or the ethicist can seek assistance from persons who do have them, but they must be present in some form if she is successfully to manage activist change.

Furthermore, any power attached to the outsider's status can be very fragile. If the ethicist does not have institutional respect, or if it is tenuous, her effectiveness can be quickly undercut if key institutional members view her as overstepping their perception of her appropriate role. Realistically, a politically oriented ethicist will routinely find herself at odds with the aims and actions of many in the hospital organization. The ethicist must find a balance, advocating structural change on Monday, focusing on microlevel clinical concerns on Thursday. If she pushes structural concerns too hard, she will be ignored or outright dismissed; if she focuses only on the micro-clinical concerns, she addresses only part of clinical encounters.

Also, while it seems clear that an adequate clinical ethics must get at root problems, there is a danger of being spread too thin, of focusing too much time, energy, and resources on political structures, thus leaving too little for effective clinical work. Balance is again critical. Further, the politically active clinical ethicist may recruit institutional allies to sometimes carry the ball. This will help ensure she does not devote too much of her resources, and her political capital, on the structural level, thus undercutting her effectiveness in the clinic and also thereby obviating the efficiency argument.

And last, while the arguments above address the problem of co-option, it still looms large.[34] The financial and status incentives attached to the job can be quite powerful, making it all too tempting to become enmeshed, to lose one's critical, outsider perspective. Thus the point of this chapter: Clinical ethicists must become politically informed, aware of and responsive to political and institutional structures and their relationship to specific clinical cases.[35] Becoming so informed can occur in part through academic training, but the model also requires a different attitude, a looking at the world through politicized lenses. Once politicized, one can no longer view (most) microlevel cases as divorced from structural problems. Thus the question becomes one of character: being willing to do the right thing, even at some personal risk.

The ethicist should also, of course, pick her fights. My own strategy is to take on one or two issues of particular importance at a time. Further, whether the focus is social or institutional should be determined by one's sentiments and by the organizational culture in which one works. For some, it would be safer and more effective to advocate social change; for others, institutional structures would be a better target.

In saying all this I am also fully aware that political activists will of course not always push the agenda with which I'm sympathetic. Leon Kass, the recently resigned chairman of the President's Council on Bioethics, became a lightning rod not just for his views on such matters as stem cell research, but for what many took to be his *advocating* for those views and thereby his politicizing of the council.[36] While I disagree with most of his conclusions and with some of his methods, I can hardly criticize Kass for attempting to achieve the ethical goals consistent with his deepest convictions. I see it instead as the job of the other members of the council to come back at him just as hard, to advocate for their convictions, and to attempt, through both ethical reasoning and political persuasion, to alter his views.

To pretend, hence, that these complex moral problems exist independently of social and political context is, in short, folly, a reality ethics consultants will have to recognize if they wish to have a genuine impact on the institutions in which they practice.

# Notes

1. Mark Aulisio and Robert Arnold, "Ethics Consultation: In the Service of Practice," *Journal of Clinical Ethics* 14, no. 4 (Winter 2003): 279.

2. Cf. Eliot Freidson, *Profession of Medicine: A Study of The Sociology of Applied Knowledge* (Chicago: University of Chicago Press, 1988), *Professionalism: The 3rd Logic* (Chicago: University of Chicago Press, 2001), and *Professional Powers* (Chicago: University of Chicago Press, 1986); Ivan Illich, *Medical Nemesis: The Expropriation of Health* (New York: Pantheon Books, 1976), and, with Irving Zola et al., *Disabling Professions* (Boston: Marion Boyars, 1978); Howard Waitzkin, *The Second Sickness* (New York: Free Press, 1983), *The Politics of Medical Encounters* (New Haven: Yale University Press, 1991), and *The Exploitation of Illness in a Capitalist Society* (Indianapolis: Bobbs-Merrill, 1974); Susan Sontag, *Illness as Metaphor* and *AIDS as Its Metaphors* (New York: Doubleday, 1990).

3. Cf. Larry Churchill, *Rationing Health Care in America: Perceptions and Principles of Justice* (South Bend, IN: University of Notre Dame Press, 1987); Daniel Callahan, *Setting Limits: Medical Goals in an Aging Society* (Washington, DC: Georgetown University Press, 1995); Robert H. Blank, *Rationing Medicine* (New York: Columbia University Press, 1990); Norman Daniels, et al., *Is Inequality Bad for Our Health?* (Boston: Beacon Press, 2000); Norman Daniels, *Benchmarks of Fairness for Health Care Reform* (New York: Oxford University Press, 1976), and *Just Health Care* (Cambridge: Cambridge University Press, 1985); Allen Buchanan et al., *From Choice to Chance: Genetics and Justice* (Cambridge: Cambridge University Press, 2000); and Allen Buchanan, *Ethics, Efficiency, and the Market* (Lanham, MD: Rowman & Littlefield, 1985).

4. Waitzkin, *The Second Sickness*, 4–5. See also Vincent Navarro, ed., *Health and Medical Care in the U.S.: A Critical Analysis* (Farmingdale, NY: Baywood Publishing, 1975). Paul Starr, in his influential *The Social Transformation of American Medicine* (New York: Basic Books, 1982), makes a similar case, using a social historian's methodology to stress the relationship between historically rooted social structures—like the emergence of the American Medical Association—and contemporary medical practice.

5. Cf. Albert Jonsen, Mark Siegler, and William Winslade, *Clinical Ethics*, 6th ed. (New York: McGraw-Hill, 2006), and John LaPuma and David Schiedermayer, *Ethics Consultation: A Practical Guide* (Boston: Jones and Bartlett Publishers, 1994). A partial exception is Richard M. Zaner, ed., *Performance, Talk, Reflection: What Is Going on in Clinical Ethics Consultation* (Dordrecht: Kluwer, 1999).

6. Waitzkin, *The Second Sickness*, 7.

7. Aulisio and Arnold, "Ethics Consultation," 277.

8. See Ludwig Wittgenstein, *Philosophical Grammar*, trans. A. J. Kenny (Berkeley: University of California Press, 1978).

9. I say "superficial" because I think US health care is committed far more to an ideology of *assent* than of *consent*. Christopher Meyers, "Cruel Choices: Autonomy and Critical Care Decision-Making," *Bioethics* 18, no. 2 (April 2004): 104–19.

10. This ideology is gradually changing, but the fight against death is still easily the predominant medical ethos.

11. See Alfred Schutz, "Some Structures of the Life-World," in *Phenomenology and Sociology*, ed. Thomas Luckmann (New York: Penguin Books, 1978): 257–74.

12. See Gaye Tuchmann, "Objectivity as Strategic Ritual: An Examination of Newsmen's Notions of Objectivity," *American Journal of Sociology* 77, no. 4 (January 1972): 660–79. See also Terry Eagleton, *Ideology* (New York: Verso, 1991), 58.

13. Schutz, "Some Structures of the Life-World," 257, 258.

14. See Eagleton, *Ideology*, 3.

15. Those mutual relationships, the ways in which each level is altered in its relation to others, are far more complex than I can give justice to here. I restrict my analysis to noting that political ideologies and organizational cultures affect, inform, are present in, and partly determine clinical ethics cases. For a more thorough discussion see Jeffrey C. Alexander et al., eds. *The Macro-Micro Link* (Berkeley: University of California Press, 1987).

16. Waitzkin, *The Politics*, 3.

17. Waitzkin, *The Politics*, 4.

18. Exceptions, interestingly enough, most often came from international commentators. Cf. "No Feeding Tubes for Me!," with comments by Richard H. Nicholson (British), Hans-Georg Koch, and Tatjana Ulshoefer and Ren-Zong Qiu, *Hastings Center Report* (International Supplement) 17, no. 3 (June 1987): 23–26. The other exception, of course, is those cases focusing on allocation of scarce resources and health care policy. Even those, though, tended to focus more on *politics* than on the *political*. Cf. Paul B. Hoffman, "How Best Shall We Serve," with comments by Mitchell T. Rabkin, Corrine Bayley, and Dan Beauchamp, *Hastings Center Report* 23, no. 2 (March–April 1993): 29–32; and "The HMO Physician's Duty to Cut Costs," with comments by Robert Veatch and Morris Collen, *Hastings Center Report* 15, no. 4 (August 1985): 13–18.

19. *Hastings Center Report* 22, no. 3 (April–May 1992): 26–27. Silverman is an emergency department physician and Dennis is an attorney; Rouse is executive director of the Mayday Fund and Director of Legal Services, Choice in Dying, Inc. This example is also revealing in that discussion of AIDS cases often has a thoroughly politicized tone, no doubt due to the politicized nature of much of the AIDS public discourse.

20. *Hastings Center Report* 10, no. 3 (June 1980): 22–24. Carson is director of the Institute for the Medical Humanities at the University of Texas Medical Branch in Galveston; Aranow (deceased) was a professor of medicine at College of Physicians and Surgeons, Columbia University. Rhoden (deceased) was a professor of law at the University of North Carolina. The case is older and thus some of the attitudes expressed in the commentary have hopefully evolved, but Bette-Jane Crigger considered it current enough to include in her 1998 compilation of such cases, *Cases in Bioethics*, 3rd ed. (New York: St. Martin's Press, 1998).

21. *Hastings Center Report* 30, no. 6 (November–December 2000): 24–25. Cotler is professor and chair of the Department of Health Sciences, California State University, Northridge. She is also clinical ethics consultant for several Southern California hospitals and nursing homes. Ganzini is director of geriatric psychiatry at the Portland Veterans Medical Center in Portland, Oregon. Cohen is codirector of the Psychiatric Consultation Service at the Bay State Medical Center in Springfield, Massachusetts.

22. See Meyers, "Cruel Choices."

23. I would also emphasize that all the issues raised in these cases are still very much present in contemporary clinical practice; for example, I still regularly struggle to get clinicians—and hospital administrators—to treat gay partners as having comparable moral rights to their heterosexual counterparts.

24. Jorge J. E. Garcia, "Philosophy in American Public Life: De Facto and De Jure," *Proceedings and Addresses of the American Philosophical Association* 72 (May 1999): 149–58. Quoted in Kathie Jenni's essay, "The Moral Responsibilities of Intellectuals," *Social Theory and Practice* 27, no. 3 (July 2001): 443.

25. Like all such issues, this one is more complex than is often portrayed. For example, given that I am regularly identified and quoted by our local press as a death penalty opponent, it seems silly and dishonest to take a neutral position on the matter in the classroom. This does not mean I do not attempt to give due credence to the opposing views, but in the end I advocate an abolitionist perspective.

26. Cf. William F. May, *Beleaguered Rulers* (Louisville, KY: Westminster John Knox Press, 2001).

27. For those who are employed full-time by the hospital and who also do not have tenure or similar job security, the following arguments apply only to the extent their institution respects and promotes academic and critical freedom.

28. I expand on this point in chapter 4.

29. I am grateful to Bill Lynn for his suggestions here.

30. I would note, however, the attorney at the hospital where I do the bulk of my work has concluded this approach is wholly consistent with legal intent. The development of next-of-kin ordering has its roots in generalities; that is generally speaking, spouses, adult children, parents, and so on, are the best surrogates. When they are not, then *both* law and ethics demand going to the (outside) person who is.

31. Christopher Meyers, "Clinical Ethics Consulting and Conflicts of Interest: Structurally Intertwined," *Hastings Center Report* 37, no. 2 (March–April 2007): 2–10.

32. Robert Veatch, "Clinical Ethics, Applied Ethics, and Theory," in *Clinical Ethics: Theory and Practice*, ed. Barry Hoffmaster, Benjamin Freedman, and Gwen Fraser (Clifton, NJ: Humana Press, 1989), 20.

33. Gerald Dopplet, "The Medical Ethicist as the Empirically Based Consultant: A Critique" (presented as a response to an earlier version of this paper at the American Philosophical Association Pacific Division Meetings, San Francisco, March 2001).

34. Dopplet and Jeffrey Paris have pushed me hard on this point, for which I am very grateful.

35. They may also call for changes to the roles of physicians, nurses, and other medical personnel to approach their work with greater political awareness, but the focus here is on clinical ethicists.

36. "'I think Leon went too far to engage himself in the politics of the topics the council considered, writing newspaper op-eds and going on the think-tank circuit,' said Arthur Caplan, chairman of the department of medical ethics at the University of Pennsylvania Medical School. In several cases, Caplan said, Kass seemed to be pushing for a consensus that would be in line with the White House's preordained views on a topic. 'I think that may have damaged some of what he tried to accomplish,' Caplan said." Rick Weiss, "Bioethics Council Head to Step Down, *Washington Post*, 9 September 2005, A6.

CHAPTER FOUR

~

# Why Do Good People
# Do Bad Things?

"To grasp why human beings act as they do, we must understand the meaning of their activity." —Anthony Giddens[1]

Every practical ethics methodology accepts that empirical facts are critical to effective analysis and consulting. Indeed, practical ethics provides the contrary to the old philosophical cliché, usually only half-jokingly told: "Never let the facts get in the way of a good theory." Practical ethics of all stripes, and especially clinical ethics, are directly dependent on a full description and understanding of the relevant facts. This is particularly true, since, as discussed above, clinical ethics problems often entail only confusion about or disagreement over facts, with little or no value conflict.

Thus what are to count as "facts" takes on critical importance. Which ones and of what sort are necessary to effective ethics consulting?

Clinical ethics largely relies on the case-study approach rooted in law and medicine. In nearly all such studies the cases are presented as a relatively simple mix of straightforward facts.[2] Little attention is given to social or institutional factors, to political or other power structures, or to professional and organizational cultures. Although case studies can certainly get at important aspects of ethical problems, as noted above, the standard method does not capture the array of factors that underlie and contribute to the dilemma.

---

Significant portions of this chapter were previously published in my article, "Institutional Culture and Individual Behavior: Creating an Ethical Environment," *Journal of Science and Engineering Ethics* 10, no. 2 (April 2004): 269–76.

Thus any emerging recommendations will touch on only part of what is actually at stake in the problem.

Robert Zussman draws attention to the importance of richer empirical analysis. Using managed care as an example, he concludes:

> What becomes critical, then, to understanding the ethical implications of managed care is . . . an understanding of the social context in which physicians make sense of and evaluate [compensation schemes]. . . . The social sciences— and sociology in particular—can lend a bit of reality to the flights of fancy that sometimes characterize the more speculative versions of philosophical medical ethics. Sociology, particularly in its ethnographic mode, may provide a method of discovery that has been slighted elsewhere.[3]

Broaden Zussman's notion of "social context" to include chapter 3's conception of "the political," and his point becomes all the more forceful. Having a political mentality is crucial, but of little value without some means for getting determinative facts, facts that include institutional beliefs and norms.

## Organizational Culture

The argument in chapter 3, though inclusive of both political and institutional structures, emphasized the former. Here I shift focus, in part because an understanding of institutional structures necessitates a different empirical method. Thus this chapter has two aims—first, to show how organizational culture develops and motivates agents' values and behavior and, second, to describe an empirical method for making sense out of that culture so as to gain a more complete understanding of the full range of facts that impact clinical ethics cases. Those analyses also reinforce the conclusion from chapter 3 that an effective prescriptivism also requires an *activist* approach.

As noted above, becoming politically informed requires mainly a process of education in political and ideological theory, along with a shift in attention and attitude. To fully appreciate *institutional* structures, though, one must acquire both a different understanding of what are to count as the relevant facts and a different means for getting at them. This is because such structures reflect broader social and political rules and norms and their *internal* reality. Institutional structures also, in turn, serve to motivate individuals' institutionally based values and behaviors, and thus are directly present in bedside ethical dilemmas. In short, all complex organizations, including health care institutions, are mini-societies. These societies develop normative cultures, ones that reflect and incorporate macrolevel sociopolitical realities while also acting upon microlevel conditions and choices. Thus, no ethical dilemma represents merely tension among conflicting moral principles or malevolent individual choices; each also instantiates the cultural norms present at the institutional and social levels.

Literature in business ethics explicitly embraces this point and is replete with discussions of organizational culture and its impact on the ethical behavior and attitudes of employees.[4] In fact the only real debate in that literature seems to be whether organizational culture has a distinct ontological status or is reducible to institutional agents.[5] Given how dominant cultural analyses are in that literature, it is surprising how little is present in bioethics, especially given the complex nature of health care institutions.[6] Indeed, few organizations have richer internal cultures than teaching hospitals, with their entrenched hierarchies, blend of professional groups, socially conferred power and status, and potential for life-or-death impact on their clients.[7]

Put another way, since all clinical ethicists agree they must have a good grasp of the facts, the organizational culture model notes that those facts must include the nature of the institutional culture and its impact on agents. That is, the ethicist's empirical understanding must go much deeper than is generally included in the shallow empiricism of the case-study model.

## Good People, Bad Actions

Why must her understanding go much deeper? So that she can answer the title of this chapter, "Why Do Good People Do Bad Things?" The question has to be asked in this way because much of ethics, both popular and professional, presumes that morally bad actions result from three sources: good people making mistakes (out of confusion or ignorance), good people having weakness of will, or bad people choosing to do evil. With this presupposition as a backdrop, the goal of practical ethics becomes finding ways to help good people avoid mistakes, to determine how to strengthen weak wills, and to establish appropriate punishment for evildoers. Theory and method, then, become tools for achieving this goal; that is, they provide principled guidance and explain when to exact retribution when such guidance fails.

Such a goal is a worthwhile start, as many ethical problems do result from error, weakness, and vice. But many also result from an organizational culture that promotes internal or prudential values at the expense of ethical ones, for example, when the culture values productivity over moral principles.[8] Within such a culture, good people will thus sometimes make "correct" choices that are nonetheless ethically problematic. That is, they will make knowledgeable choices, they will do so with strength of character and virtuously, and yet these choices will be unethical.

This claim is admittedly counterintuitive. How can it be that good people make correct choices that are nonetheless unethical? The question has to be answered in two parts. First, why are the choices "unethical"? And, second, if they are, how can they nonetheless be "correct"? The first part is relatively easy: They are unethical because they violate accepted moral principles or produce ethically undesirable outcomes, at least as the choices are seen from outside the organization.

## Setting the Values

The "outside the organization" caveat points to the answer to the second part: Persons within the organization make choices consistent with its cultural values—with its norms, its goals, its beliefs—and because of this consistency the choices are organizationally "correct," even when they do not align with broader moral principles. In its stronger form, such consistency becomes a mindset, a filter through which participants view their world. And it does more than simply motivate certain attitudes; it also works to create a conceptual scheme. As noted above, Patricia Werhane describes and analyzes the nature and importance of organizational culture and explains the process as follows:

> We all perceive, frame, and interact with the world through a conceptual scheme modified by a set of perspectives or mental models. Putting the point metaphorically, we each run our "camera" of the world through certain selective mechanisms: intentions, interests, desires, points of view, or biases, all of which work as selective and restrictive filters. We each have what I call our own metaphysical movies of the world, because they entail projections of one's perspective on the given data of experience.[9]

These schemes, especially when they are rooted in a powerful group culture, significantly contribute to how agents perceive problems, how they categorize them, how they understand and ascribe value, and when and how they act. As Robert Willmott puts it, organizational cultures represent "distinct, irreducible strata of reality, possessing relational causal properties of their own, which react back upon their progenitors to modify, constrain or enable human agency."[10] Dennis Gioia, the Ford manager responsible for making the recommendation not to recall the Pinto despite the car's history of devastating fires following minor accidents, describes Ford's culture in his memoir of those events:

> My own schematized . . . knowledge influenced me to perceive recall issues in terms of the prevailing decision environment and to *unconsciously overlook* key features of the Pinto case, mainly because they did not fit an existing script. Al-

though the outcomes of the case carry retrospectively obvious ethical overtones, the schemas driving my perceptions and actions precluded consideration of the issues in ethical terms because the scripts did not include ethical dimensions.[11]

This description reveals why traditional accountability ascription, that is, why appeal to evil intent, weakness of will, or error is inadequate. By all accounts Gioia was hardly a vicious person; his narrative does not fit weakness of will, which assumes the agent knows better but gives in to temptation. And his choices were anything but ignorant—he had all the relevant facts at his disposal. In short, he was a reasonably virtuous, informed person who nonetheless did bad things. The key to seeing why this follows is present in Gioia's statement that he "unconsciously overlook[ed] key features" of the case. It is not that he *chose* to set those aside or that in a cowardly fashion he refused to broach them with his superior; rather, *he literally did not see them.* He was caught up in the organizational script or ethos.

## Capturing the Ethos

Difficult to describe, an ethos is a complex, systematic, value-based structure that in large part determines what is internally accepted as institutionally appropriate ethical behavior; that is, it is the value-based foundation of an organizational culture. As Max Stackhouse describes it, "[A]n ethos . . . is the subtle web of values, meanings, purposes, expectations, obligations, and legitimations that constitutes the operating norms of a culture."[12] As such, an institutional ethos is a mix of macrolevel political structures and institutional culture, and microlevel personal beliefs and values.

For ethicists, the most relevant aspects of these include the following:

1. Formal and informal methods of rewarding and punishing. These comprise formal disciplinary actions, along with the less obvious informal processes like work assignments, public versus private criticism, and the extent to which superiors engage a subordinate in relaxed social conversation or shared meals.
2. The relationship between what is said, especially publicly, and what is done, especially privately. This factor in institutional culture is among the more telling, and it is relatively easy to discern: Do agents' deeds match their words? It is particularly important to test the match of words and actions in institutional power brokers, since their behavior establishes, through role modeling, what the institution will count as acceptable conduct.

3. Power relationships. To whom does the group defer? Who has the final word? Who verbally interrupts whom? Who is nearly always referred to by professional title and who are those who do not follow this norm? How does body language reveal power (e.g., Who sits first? Who engages in other activities, like reading a chart, while others speak? Who walks in the front in groups?)?

These elements are explicitly present in hospital policies, leadership charts, and obvious expressions of deference, all of which are cognitively realized by decisional participants, even if they are not always explicitly present in participants' analyses and decision-making. And, as apparent, they do not require any particularly special observational skill by the ethicist. She can retain her position as an outsider, watching, paying close attention and thereby coming to better understand the institutional ethos and its motivational force. The basic methodological requirements are as simple as relevant and informed interest, a shift in focus (adding observation to analysis), and a willingness to commit the time.

They are also *implicitly* present in subtle expressions of institutional values, in the ways those with power express social approval, ranging from the giving of promotions to invitations to lunch or for drinks, to the "nudge-nudge, wink-wink" forms of body language. Key here is the relationship between what managers say is of value and what they actually reinforce, combined with the recognition that according to most accounts of organizational theory, it is the implicit and subtle processes that most effectively establish organizational culture. Humans respond more to behavioral reinforcement than to verbal rules and policies.

Take, for example, the debacle involving Jayson Blair and the *New York Times*, in which it was discovered that Blair, a hot young star at the nation's leading newspaper, had plagiarized (or made up) many of his news stories. You can be sure editors at the *Times* verbally extol the value of honest and accurate reporting. Yet, despite mounting evidence of problems, they also regularly, and preferentially, treated Blair to lunch and drinks and gave him plum assignments. As was widely discussed among journalists and social critics, racial factors no doubt contributed to this unusual treatment (Blair is African American); but the important point here is that editors reinforced his unethical practices through their approval behavior, even though, again, they verbally condemned such practices.

Often, maybe most often, the subtle reinforcement is negative, and again ranges from simple body language (e.g., physically turning away from someone) to communication style (e.g., interrupting speakers, not answering questions) to chastising. An example of this occurred during the debate over space shuttle Challenger's O-rings. Morton Thiokol's Jerry Mason responded to the cold-weather fears of his vice president of engineering, Robert Lund, by saying, "[T]ake off [your] engineering hat and put on [your] management hat."[13] With that simple statement, Mason effectively established the organization's fundamental cultural norm, recreated Lund's corporate script, and set the stage for disaster.

## Different Meanings

At a deeper level, though, the organizational ethos is considerably more complex and subtle. The observer is not just looking for explicit rules, power and turf, or even for body language and social approval; she is also trying to understand how the ethos determines institutionally grounded *meaning*. On this view, key ethical concepts, like autonomy, futility, and informed consent, derive their meaning in large part through the organizational culture. Thus it is possible, even likely, that two persons from significantly different organizational cultures (e.g., academic philosophy and institutional medicine) can use the same terms but mean something almost entirely different and thus end up talking past one another. The differences may be minor and of little consequence, or major with profound implications for patient care.

For example, when philosophers speak of promoting autonomy, they usually mean a complex notion of moral agency, choosing a conception of the good, acting according to a life plan.[14] By contrast, for most physicians autonomy generally means *assent*. That is, when a patient "autonomously" accedes to or goes along with a recommended treatment plan, most physicians believe she has thereby expressed an autonomous choice. The much richer notions of personal integrity, consistency, and accountability so present in the philosophical conception are at least greatly downplayed, if not altogether absent from the medical understanding, an understanding directly informed by institutional and professional cultures.[15] In these medical cultures, more often than not, patient acquiescence to physician authority is highly preferred over genuine autonomy, given that the latter typically slows down the medical encounter and often creates unwanted complications for the physician.

Hence I can have a seemingly clear and coherent conversation with a resident in which we agree that it is important to promote patient autonomy, walk away pleased in our agreement, and yet in critical respects have fundamentally misunderstood one another. Thus when she goes off to implement a recommendation to respect or promote patient autonomy, the resident will act in ways substantially different than intended in the proffered advice.

It is neither reasonable nor realistic to expect the resident to think like a philosopher, to have the richer, more complex conception of autonomy. Thus if she and I are going to reach genuine agreement, and since I have been hired to provide the ethics advice, even expertise, it becomes my obligation to acquire a sufficiently rich understanding of *her* culture and semantics. This is not just a question of philosophers and clinicians using different technical terminology; it is a problem of different *conceptual schemes*.

### Worldviews

The metaphysics and epistemology at work here—summarized by Calvin Morrill and Gary Fine as, "we know things by their meanings, . . . meanings are created through social interaction, and . . . meanings change through interaction"[16]—have their roots in twentieth-century phenomenological and Wittgensteinian life-world and forms of life philosophy.[17] Tying together these otherwise diverse views is the conclusion that to get at the meaning of actions, beliefs, and attitudes, one must get at the intersubjectively constituted structure of beliefs and rules that define cultures and institutions and that thus also serve to motivate and guide behaviors within them.

The philosophical literature on this topic could fill a library, and there is anything but consensus on how meaning is established and maintained.[18] Without stepping too deep into that fray, I want to make the relatively uncontroversial claim that how terms are used—the role they play in organizing and making sense of complex social structures and relationships—helps determine agents' meaningful understanding of them.

Thus, to stick with the example, what "autonomy" means to a third-year resident differs from what it means for an academic philosopher, which differs from what it means for a lawyer, for an ethicist, for a patient, and so on. Again, the meaning of terms is largely defined by the social and institutional purposes they serve, and thus in order to avoid the "talking past" problem noted above, ethicists need a fuller understanding of those social and institutional purposes, of the motivating ethos.

Unfortunately, unlike the more readily apparent explicit rules, power relationships, and defined turf discussed above, the ethos is reflected in how terms are *used*, as opposed to how they are formally defined, and thus it is better revealed in behavior and in responses to problems and conflict. Just as ideologies and social frameworks create macrolevel political structures, so an institutional ethos creates organizational meaning structures. Hubert Dreyfus calls these structures "primordial" and the knowledge institutional members have, "practical understanding." Such understanding, he says, is holistic in an entirely different way from theoretical understanding. Although practical understanding—everyday coping with things and people—involves explicit beliefs and hypotheses, these can only be meaningful in specific contexts and against a background of shared practices. And just as we learn to swim without consciously or unconsciously acquiring a theory of swimming, we acquire these social background practices by being brought up in them.[19]

Take another example: In my work with ICU residents I stress the now-standard line that informed consent is much more than a signature on a form, that it is a process intended both to confirm genuine consent and to keep often frightened and alienated patients informed about routine goings-on (e.g., clinical exams, blood draws, and various other pokings and proddings). I include in this discussion procedures that generally do not require formal consent but that are nonetheless emotionally disruptive for patients, such as CT scans without contrast. This procedure, though, is so common residents tend to treat it as not worthy of a standard informed consent conversation. Convincing them otherwise is usually not a tough sell; most residents come quickly to appreciate how such conversations, though not technically required by law or hospital policy, can do much to relieve patients' anxiety. After our conversation, residents thus pledge they will make the effort to keep patients so informed.

Despite these assurances, I have repeatedly watched technicians come in, gather up, and wheel off clearly startled and confused patients who have no idea where they are going and little clue about even what a CT scan is or does.[20] Some of those confusions are often, though not always, cleared up once the patient arrives in radiology, but even so, it is then too late to relieve the anxiety caused by the initial unexplained disruption.

On the standard case-study approach, the facts would be described just as above and the ethicist would chastise the resident for being insensitive, even callous. On an organizational culture account, however, additional facts would be included, the first two of which are broadly applicable to the medical profession, the last two specific to the particular institution. While these added details give only a partial picture of relevant professional and institutional culture, they still provide more information than is characteristically provided in the case-study method.

1. These are horribly overstressed residents who resent and thus avoid additional work that is not mandated either by law or by a person who holds genuine authority.

2. Medical residents fall fairly low on the medical totem pole and are regularly required to engage a wide range of undesirable tasks. They thus quickly learn to avoid extra work or to shuffle it off to other unfortunates further down the line, all while giving higher-ups every assurance that the requested task will be competently handled.

3. Although I have good standing in the institution and am regularly called upon to assist in difficult cases, residents know that I have limited institutional authority. Except in egregious cases, I can neither reward nor punish and thus my exhortations can usually be ignored without consequence.

4. The hospital's then-director of the ICU had a paternal attitude toward patients and thus insisted residents not "overly burden them" with potentially fearful information. But because she did not always do a good job of teaching residents how to distinguish anxiety-*inducing* from anxiety-*relieving* information, they tended to err on the side of (their) safety, concluding that too little is better than too much.

These additional facts are clearly relevant to the ethicist's analysis and subsequent recommendations. They provide a better understanding of the residents' behavior: If residents are insensitive or callous, they are nonetheless still within their cultural norm, a fact that should temper any critique directed at individuals. Wendy Carlton nicely captures this point: "The obliqueness of physician attention to . . . ethical issues is not a function of stupidity or ignorance; . . . it is founded on institutional constraints which reinforce certain kinds of behavior that have been elicited and rewarded throughout professional training."[21]

Having this cultural knowledge also helps to focus the ethicist's efforts at enhancing ethical behavior. To be most effective, she needs to pursue a number of new strategies: She should learn to be sufficiently savvy to hollow assurances, she should concentrate on giving residents time-constrained methods for providing information, she should work to increase her own institutional authority, and she should try to encourage attending physicians to give residents better tools for discriminating among more and less important kinds of information and to assist her in the teaching of this. That is, as I stressed in chapter 3, her prescriptive approach must also be an activist approach, actively striving to alter professional and institutional structures that consistently contribute to ethical lapses.

Would these conclusions emerge from the empirically shallow case-study method? Possibly, but not likely. Think back to the initially narrow case descriptions and analyses discussed in chapter 3. A more complete discussion requires that one go deeper, to the subtle processes of behavior determinants. As Richard Zaner puts it, in "institutional contexts such as hospitals and medical units . . . the 'unspoken' recipes of action govern quite as much as the written codes and even more powerfully."[22] Those unspoken recipes make up the heart of the organizational culture, and thus the ethicist, if she is genuinely going to understand what is at work in a given dilemma, must have a sufficiently rich grasp of that culture.

Hence the import of a nuanced empirical methodology: The practices of working professionals are learned skills and are displayed through *behavior* far more clearly than through an analysis of written rules. Again, Dreyfus: "[A]greement in judgments means agreement in what people *do* and *say*, not what they *believe*."[23] For an outsider thus to come truly to understand institutional practices, she must engage in "prolonged interaction, the result [of which] is what Heidegger calls 'finding a footing' and Wittgenstein refers to as 'finding one's way about.'"[24] That understanding must also, then, find its way into the ethicist's attempts to create a more ethical environment. Such attempts can occur through work with individuals, but to be most effective, they must also be directed at professional and organizational norms.

## Understanding the Culture

Noting, however, that organizational culture has a powerful influence over members' ethical behavior says nothing about how one should go about accessing it. What are the best ways of doing so, especially for philosophers with almost no training in empirical methodology?

Discovering much of what serves to define organizational culture—for example, formal and informal rules, institutional policies, hierarchical pecking order, mission statements, company newsletters—does not require special training, but rather a shift in attention. The ethicist needs to be as much an observer as an advisor.[25] For example, she should participate in rounds, but should do so to learn as well as to consult. She should seek membership on hospital committees (bioethics, obviously, but also institutional review board, patient rights, etc.), again observing intently. She should occasionally take meals in the hospital (staff) cafeteria. She should try to arrange to shadow a resident for a couple of thirty-six-hour shifts or follow a member of the faculty for a week. And she should attend hospital and department functions, for instance, annual meetings and awards ceremonies. In all this she is attempting to see the organization as participants do, to appreciate how explicit institutional norms and pressures impact participants' perceptions of genuine options and thereby also to better understand motivations behind their eventual choices.

## Ethnography

If, however, she wishes an even more sophisticated grasp of the culture, not just of the explicit rules, norms, and power structures, but at a level adequate to identify and eventually to critically analyze the institutional practices that define normative meaning, she also needs a sufficiently sophisticated empirical method. Of the various ones available, the one best able to address the problem of differing semantics is ethnography, broadly understood here to include internal observation, ethnomethodology, and linguistic analysis.[26]

Although hardly a new method—scholars from sociology,[27] anthropology,[28] and those doing non-discipline-specific practical ethics[29] have defended variants of it for years—appeals to an ethnographic approach are virtually nonexistent in the philosophical ethics literature.[30] As traditionally conceived, ethics theory attempts to meld coherent views of metaphysics, epistemology, and action theory so as to give a better understanding of what it means to be a moral human being and to provide broad guideposts for decision-making. By contrast, strict ethnography strives to be descriptive only. It attempts to discern the structure of cultures, institutions, and practices, and, when successful, it also often produces a better understanding of motivations for human behavior. But it strives for neutrality on the part of the observer.[31] While ethnographers gain a richer understanding of and sometimes even acquire the values of the culture under study, they almost never *evaluate* those values.[32] My recommended approach is thus a melding of this richly complex empiricism with a critically evaluative, politically informed, prescriptive clinical ethics.

Controversial even within its home disciplines—sociology and anthropology—ethnography is the subject of extensive critical literature.[33] Susan E. Kelly et al. give the following definition: "Ethnographic methods provide 'thick' or dense descriptions of ongoing social processes and insight into the meaning of actions and events from a participant's point of view."[34] In basic terms, the goal of ethnography is to understand the meaning of activities from an internal perspective, from the inside out. By becoming sufficiently immersed in the studied culture's conceptual scheme as to be conversant in it, one can, to recall this chapter's epigraph, get at the "meaning of the activity"—the norms, rules, values, and unstated codes of behavior that underlie the apparent facts.

Although the philosophically trained ethicist cannot be expected to be a true ethnographer, she can gain much by concentrating on the institutional establishment of meaning as this is revealed, for example, in power asymmetric conversation (e.g., attending/resident, physician/nurse, physician/patient). These conversations establish the rules, both formal and informal, that dictate what counts as the meaningful use of terms and thus of what passes for institutionally accepted, or desired, conduct. Furthermore, because there is already a rich body of ethnographic literature on medicine, much of it politically informed, the ethicist has key guideposts laid out.[35] That is, she can look for patterns—of power, of ideology, and of meaning—already identified by persons trained in the relevant skills.

## Different Methods

I grant that the empirical method I recommend here requires a substantial alteration of how the clinical ethicist thinks of her work. It also requires, if to a lesser extent, the acquisition of new methodological skills. Do the resulting benefits justify the change? The remainder of this chapter will argue that it does. I want first, however, to move past a common sort of confusion associated with ethnography, as exemplified by Raanan Gillon's comments in an editorial in the *Journal of Medical Ethics*:

> Even if the methodology is sociologically sound and the results are accurate, what is the ethical significance of empirical findings? . . . There is a fundamental philosophical criticism of such empirical studies, which is that even if 100 percent of a sample of people studied were found to think and act in a particular way this would not necessarily help one to decide whether their thoughts and actions were morally justifiable.[36]

If all ethnography did was give us the equivalent of a sample polling, if all it did was tell us *that* persons think and act in a certain way, it would still be of value since this would add to the pool of important facts upon which good practical ethics relies. Furthermore, ethnography goes beyond the "that" of persons' decisions to capture, as much as possible, the "why." Granted, none of this is sufficient to a politically informed, prescriptive clinical ethics; the ethicist must also engage the philosophical, conceptual, and theoretical work described in the preceding chapters. But surely the more sophisticated her empirical base, the better will the ethicist be in her evaluative tasks.

Because ethnography sees ethical meanings and behavior as intersubjectively created and maintained, a key part of the "why" is the background structure of rules and attitudes that define the organization. These rules are generally implicit rather than explicit, generated by subtle forms of reinforcement; as such, they are often beyond even the cognitive and conceptual grasp of the practitioner.[37] The rules become part of her lived practice, of her habitual way of thinking, making decisions, and acting. This is why an ethnographic method has distinct advantages over other forms of data gathering, especially over the limiting case studies so prevalent in clinical ethics. A close analysis of the institutional ethos as it is locally lived and practiced reveals motivational forces of which practitioners may not even be cognitively aware.

An example will again help. The ethics committee was called to evaluate a physician's withdrawal of treatment recommendation. The patient was in a persistent vegetative state (PVS) with no hope of recovery, subsequent to a massive hemorrhagic stroke (and myriad other ailments). The patient's surrogate, however, stated that a PVS was consistent with the patient's minimally acceptable quality of life, as per, she said, repeated conversations prior to the stroke. The attending physician, who in this and previous conversations supported an "achievement of goals" definition of futile treatment, nonetheless repeatedly insisted that continuing dialysis was futile, even though he acknowledged that such treatment would achieve the patient's desired goal, sustained life, and thus by definition was *not* futile. The case's real topic centered on whether a persistent vegetative state is in fact a desirable goal, but the physician insisted on pushing what was neither a conceptually nor an ethically sound option—that futility could be used as an "out" to justify withdrawing treatment.

While on the standard approach the physician's actions appear irrational, even contradictory, on an ethnographic analysis his behavior can be reasonably interpreted as wholly consistent with a range of social, professional, and institutional structures: direct and indirect pressures from hospital administration and third-party payers to limit treatment on "hopeless" patients; a professional culture that emphasizes healing to the extent that it creates a reluctance to devote much effort on a patient one cannot cure; a fear that the longer the patient remains hospitalized the more likely it is the physician (and others) would feel he somehow failed the patient; the stated unwillingness by the physician (and others in the group) to trust fully a poor and poorly educated surrogate (about whom suspicion was expressed because she was authorized to handle the patient's financial accounts, including Social Security income); and the many other subtle pressures from nurses, respiratory therapists, social workers, medical students who generally want to avoid terminal cases. In short, the very *meaning* of "futility" was, for the physician, determined as much, even more, by his professional and institutional ethos as by careful conceptual analysis.

Recognizing this difference significantly alters how the physician, and the case as a whole, should be approached so as to effect the ethically best outcome. He essentially needed approval from persons of at least comparable institutional power that continued treatment was consistent with organizational norms. Thus I sought out such approval (from the institution's medical director) and when that was given, the attending readily backed off. The committee then focused on the surrogate's understanding of the patient's wishes regarding quality of life. Through such discussions the surrogate eventually affirmed that such a life was probably not what the patient would wish for, a supportive care order was given, and the patient died within days.

The same result may well have been achieved using the standard method, but it almost certainly would have involved greater conflict between physician and surrogate; that is, the physician would simply have asserted his authority and declared treatment futile. Although this approach would have been "effective," it also would have been significantly more harmful for all involved, as it would have *imposed*, rather than *achieved*, the outcome. The case thus shows how even the clearest understanding of principles and concepts must also align with actual facts, including participants' motivational forces. All involved agreed autonomy and beneficence were the principles most at stake. All also agreed on how to define futile treatment and on the superficially understood presentation of the facts. What was thus also needed was the *deeper* set of facts, accessible only through a politically informed, organizationally aware, ethnographic explication. Having this, and having the right institutional contacts, allowed the conversation to shift so as to achieve everyone's desired outcome in a way that was also mutually supportive.

There is a second reason why an ethnographic approach to clinical ethics methodology is important. When the ethicist is truly an outsider, with little understanding of, and even less appreciation for, life in the clinical trenches, she will necessarily bring an outside-in approach to her work. That is, she will use an external perspective to determine what problems exist in a given enterprise, rather than going in and discerning what practitioners judge to be problematic. Those in the trenches often rightly perceive this approach as both arrogant and uninformed. As Zaner notes,

> [D]espite their efforts to work alongside physicians . . . philosophers involved [in a five-year collaborative project] came to the gloomy conclusion that, "like midwives, philosophers may be dismissed by physicians as amateurish invaders of well-governed territory. Professionals resent those who do not accept the technical routines by which professional practice is defined and justified."[38]

An ethnographic approach, by contrast, provides both enriched understanding and enhanced appreciation for the lives and choices of working practitioners; it enhances the ethicist's ability to walk in clinicians' shoes.

Third, since the standard approach devotes so much attention to the individual, it tends to ignore the extent to which individuals and their actions are grounded in a social context, with its reinforcing norms and values.[39] This emphasis on discrete individuals making independent autonomous choices draws particular criticism from Barry Hoffmaster: "Perhaps the most prominent tenet of orthodox medical ethics is its individualism, manifested by the field's conspicuous preoccupation with the notion of autonomy," a tenet, he rightly concludes, that "does not capture the realities of clinical practice."[40] Kathy Charmaz and Virginia Olesen are similarly critical:

> Ethnographic research in medical ethics has revealed the limitations of the dominant philosophical model. Its radical individualism makes collective forces and allegiances invisible and reduces challenges to the institution of medicine to requests for more thorough individual reasoning. . . . [Traditional] medical ethicists do not see the institutional and interactive roots of their moral concepts and categories. They remain unaware of how social constraints and power arrangements affect their moral vocabularies and ethical decisions.[41]

Fundamental to an ethnographic approach, by contrast, is the belief that because core meanings are defined through intersubjective organizational culture, many unethical behaviors are not the product of independent autonomous choices but instead result from factors endemic to the very structure of the institution. As such, the causes go unnoticed, except in the most egregious examples, because they are seen to be normal business, how things are done, part of the *given*.

The standard approach, alternatively, all too often promotes the "bad apple" mentality, that is, unethical occurrences are the result of an occasional bad apple or of virtuous individuals who have a rare weakness of will. When one perceives ethical problems in this light, the solution is simple: Cull the unscrupulous or bolster the morally weak. Having accomplished this when the circumstances demand, all may return to work secure in the sanctity of their endeavors. The ethos model, on the other hand, recognizes that while bad apples and weakness of will surely exist, ethicists must go beyond these to notice that the structures of the organizational culture produce a climate conducive to, even encouraging of, unethical choices.[42] The model thus realizes that persons of good will and strength of character, who have a rich and thorough understanding of key ethical concepts, will sometimes make choices that are both wholly consistent with organizational norms and also nonetheless unethical. Because the standard approach, as Bruce Jennings argues, does not pay sufficient "attention to the ways in which struggling with

a problem or acting within a certain pattern of constraints or power relationships can actually transform the moral perception and understanding of
agents," it misses how resulting choices emerge from that transformation.[43]
Thus, Jennings concludes, "[A]n understanding of the way moral notions are
embedded in social practices—and of how moral perception, understanding
and aspiration can be transformed by conduct within those practices and
structures—is essential to the development of an adequate moral philosophy."[44] It is also, I hope I have shown, essential to ethicists' prescriptive
analyses and recommendations.

## Addressing the Culture

None of this is meant to preclude the possibility of independent moral evaluation and decision-making. While culture is a powerful force, it is not a determining one; individual decision-making, and thus individual accountability, is still fundamental to organizational ethics. Hence individuals need a
means of breaking outside the conceptual scheme and acting instead on
moral principles. Werhane describes the process of such breaking out as using "moral imagination" by which one engages "in a critical perspective on
oneself, one's activities, one's behavior . . . one's situation," and one's organizational script.[45] Being caught up in the script is an explanation, but not an
excuse; with an ethical commitment, and with help, one can employ moral
imagination.

The outside ethicist can be the best source for that help. In organizations
with powerful cultures, like hospitals, it is often unreasonable to expect individuals, wholly on their own, to engage in the necessary degree of moral
imagination. The culture becomes too integral a part of their identity; to a
great degree professionals *define themselves* via that culture. Thus to ask them
to be able to break outside the culture—to see the alternatives and then to
act accordingly—is in too many cases not realistic.

Enter the ethicist, who, with her different scheme, can help clinicians
break out, see alternative ways of considering problems, and explore alternative actions.[46] These skills are all part of standard ethics training in problem
evaluation, values clarification, conceptual analysis, and complex reasoning.
To be most successful at this kind of assistance, ethicists must have two additional qualifications.

They must, again, understand the institutional ethos. They must be able
to discern how it performs, how it defines values, reinforces behavior, privi-
leges some beliefs and actions while condemning others, and so on. They
must be able to speak the organizational language and to appreciate employees'

trials and tribulations. They must, again quoting Dreyfus, be able to "find [their] way about" the organization.

This leads, though, to the second qualification: The effective ethicist will become conversant in the culture without becoming immersed in it. That is, she must continue to be an outsider, or at least enough of one as not to be caught up in the script. To be able to evaluate and criticize an organization and the behavior of its employees, one must be able to make explicit the web of beliefs, values, and norms present in organizational culture and practice. The more one is immersed in the script, the less able one is to engage in the moral imagination necessary to effectively critique it when it promotes ethically problematic behavior. The ethicist too immersed in the script cannot achieve one of her key functions—to provide an objective critique of organizational norms and concomitant behavior. That is, as per the arguments in chapter 3, the ethicist becomes co-opted.

Two final recommendations emerge. First, ethics consulting should never be a full-time job; ideally, the ethicist's primary occupation and source of income will lie elsewhere, for example, in private consulting firms or academia.[47] Inculturation into the institutional ethos and co-option, while still a threat, are on this model far less likely.

Second, practical ethics educational programs, especially those in philosophy, must pay far greater attention to empirical skills and methods.[48] While such programs increasingly realize the importance of empirical investigations, few provide the necessary techniques, no doubt in largest part because program faculty do not know them. These programs should thus consider requiring students to go outside the department—to sociology, cultural anthropology, or political science—to take necessary courses.

## Conclusion

The effective clinical ethicist, thus, must be well trained in analysis and theory; she must have the right disposition for this often traumatic work; she must see the world through a politicized lens; and she must have an empirical methodology adequate to the task of determining the organizational ethos. And she must be both an insider and an outsider, that is, immersed enough in the ethos to be able to see its impact on ethical choices, but also enough of an outsider to be able to provide genuinely critical commentary.

In short, this is demanding, difficult, and consuming work. But when done well, it is also very gratifying and of genuine help to people facing agonizing decisions. In other words, clinical ethicists may in fact be worth more than Feng Shui counselors and aroma therapists.

# Notes

1. "Hermeneutics and Social Theory," in *Hermeneutics: Questions and Prospects*, ed. Gary Shapiro and Alan Sica (Amherst: University of Massachusetts Press, 1984), 218.

2. There are any number of case-study compilations in bioethics. Three of the better ones are Bette-Jane Crigger, *Cases in Bioethics*, 3rd ed. (New York: St. Martin's Press, 1998); Gregory Pence, *Classic Cases in Medical Ethics*, 3rd ed. (New York: McGraw-Hill, 2000); and John Thomas and Wilfrid Waluchow, *Well and Good: A Case Study Approach to Biomedical Ethics*, 3rd ed. (Orchard Park, NY: Broadview Press, 1998). All three include more background and analysis but still leave out the effects of professional or organizational culture.

3. Robert Zussman, "The Contributions of Sociology to Medical Ethics," *Hastings Center Report* 30, no. 1 (January–February 2000): 9, 11. Zussman is an ethnographer and author of *Intensive Care: Medical Ethics and the Medical Profession* (Chicago: University of Chicago Press, 1992). In the same issue James Lindemann Nelson also makes a somewhat less direct case for the importance of a rich empirical method: "Moral Teachings from Unexpected Quarters: Lessons for Bioethics from the Social Sciences and Managed Care," 12–17.

4. See Scott Vitell and Saviour Nwachukwu, "The Influence of Corporate Culture on Managerial Ethical Judgments," *Journal of Business Ethics* 16, no. 8 (June 1997): 757–76; James A. Benson and David L. Ross, "Sundstrand: A Case Study in Transformation of Cultural Ethics," *Journal of Business Ethics* 17, no. 4 (October 1998): 1517–27; Vincent di Norcia, "An Enterprise/Organization Ethic," *Business and Professional Ethics Journal* 7, nos. 3–4 (Fall–Winter 1988): 61–79; and James A. Waters and Frederick Bird, "The Moral Dimension of Organizational Culture," *Journal of Business Ethics* 6 (January 1987): 15–22.

5. See Robert Willmott, "Structure, Culture, and Agency: Rejecting the Current Orthodoxy of Organisation Theory," *Journal for the Theory of Social Behaviour* 27, no. 1 (January 1997): 93–123.

6. If conference presentations are an accurate indication, however, there appears to be a surging interest in this topic, in part motivated by Patricia Werhane's important work. For example, at the 2002 meetings of the Association of Practical and Professional Ethics (APPE) there were four presentations on ethics and health care organizations and Werhane gave the keynote address at the 2006 APPE meetings.

7. See Charles L. Bosk, *Forgive and Remember* (Chicago: University of Chicago Press, 1981), and Barbara Katz Rothman, *In Labor: Women and Power in the Birthplace* (New York: W. W. Norton, 1982). For an account of the medical profession's history and culture see Paul Starr, *The Social Transformation of American Medicine* (New York: Basic Books, 1982).

8. See Michael Davis, "Better Communication Between Engineers and Managers: Some Ways to Prevent Many Ethically Hard Choices," *Science and Engineering Ethics* 3, no. 2 (April 1997): 171–212.

9. Patricia Werhane, *Moral Imagination and Management Decision-making* (New York: Oxford, 1999), 49.

10. Willmott, "Structure, Culture, and Agency," 93. One of Willmott's principal concerns in this article is to address whether organizational culture is ontologically distinct.

11. Werhane, *Moral Imagination*, 56, italics added.

12. Max Stackhouse, *Ethics and the Urban Ethos: An Essay in Social Theory and Theological Reconstruction* (Boston: Beacon Press, 1972), 5.

13. Werhane, *Moral Imagination*, 49.

14. Cf. Tom Beauchamp and James Childress, *Principles of Biomedical Ethics*, 5th ed. (New York: Oxford University Press, 2001); Carl Schneider, *The Practice of Autonomy: Patients, Doctors, and Medical Decisions* (New York: Oxford University Press, 1998); Gerald Dworkin, *The Theory and Practice of Autonomy* (Cambridge: Cambridge University Press, 1988); B. H. Levi, *Respecting Patient Autonomy* (Urbana: University of Illinois Press, 1999); L. Haworth, *Autonomy: An Essay in Philosophical Psychology and Ethics* (New Haven, CT: Yale University Press, 1986); and Thomas May, *Autonomy, Authority, and Moral Responsibility* (London: Kluwer Academic Publishers, 1998).

15. Christopher Meyers, "Cruel Choices: Autonomy and Critical Care Decision-Making," *Bioethics* 18, no. 2 (April 2004): 104–19.

16. Calvin Morrill and Gary Alan Fine, "Ethnographic Contributions to Organizational Sociology," *Sociological Methods and Research* 25, no. 4 (May 1997): 428, quoting Herbert Blumer. I do not claim here that all meaning is wholly defined intersubjectively but that social processes in large part determine the meaning of events and activities, especially those with ethical import.

17. For comparative summaries of these views see Nicholas Gier, *Wittgenstein and Phenomenology* (Albany: State University of New York Press, 1981), and Richard Rorty, *Philosophy and the Mirror of Nature* (Princeton: Princeton University Press, 1979).

18. There is not even consensus on what "meaning" means!

19. Hubert Dreyfus, "Holism and Hermeneutics," *Review of Metaphysics* 34, no. 1 (September 1980), 7. The entire issue is devoted to philosophical hermeneutics, with articles by Charles Taylor, Richard Rorty, Paul Weiss, and others.

20. Again, CT scans are just one example; similar reactions are common with blood draws, X-rays, respiratory therapy, and so forth.

21. Wendy Carlton, *"In Our Professional Opinion . . .": The Primacy of Clinical Judgment over Moral Choice* (Notre Dame, IN: University of Notre Dame Press, 1978), 4.

22. Richard Zaner, *Ethics and the Clinical Encounter* (Englewood Cliffs, NJ: Prentice Hall, 1980), 31.

23. Dreyfus, "Holism and Hermeneutics," 12.

24. Dreyfus, "Holism and Hermeneutics," 12.

25. For a discussion of observational methodology see Karl E. Weick, "Systematic Observational Methods," in *The Handbook of Social Psychology*, ed. Gardner Lindzey and Elliot Aronson (Reading, MA: Addison-Wesley, 1968), 357–451.

26. For a more thorough account of ethnography and its various guises, see Virginia Olesen, "At Work in the Field(s) of Ethnography" (book review), *Journal of Contemporary Ethnography* 26, no. 4 (January 1998): 511–15; Kathy Charmaz and Virginia Olesen, "Ethnographic Research in Medical Sociology: Its Foci and Distinctive Contributions," *Sociological Methods and Research* 25, no. 4 (May 1997): 452–94; and Morrill and Fine, "Ethnographic Contributions," 424–51.

27. Cf. Morrill and Fine, "Ethnographic Contributions." See also, in the same journal and issue, Charmaz and Olesen, "Ethnographic Research."

28. Cf. George Weisz, ed., *Social Science Perspectives on Medical Ethics* (Philadelphia: University of Pennsylvania Press, 1990), especially the articles by Renee Fox, "The Evolution of American Bioethics: A Sociological Perspective," 201–17, and Richard Lieban, "Medical Anthropology and the Comparative Study of Medical Ethics," 221–39.

29. Cf. Barry Hoffmaster, "Can Ethnography Save the Life of Medical Ethics?" *Social Science and Medicine* 35, no. 12 (1992): 1421–31; David W. Robertson, "Ethical Theory, Ethnography, and Differences Between Doctors and Nurses in Approaches to Patient Care," *Journal of Medical Ethics* 22 (October 1996): 292–99 (see also the editorial by Raanan Gillon, in the same issue, "Ethnography, Medical Practice, and Moral Reflective Equilibrium," 259–60); Bette-Jane Crigger, "Bioethnography: Fieldwork in the Lands of Medical Ethics," *Medical Anthropology Quarterly* 9, no. 3 (September 1995): 400–417; and Bruce Jennings, "Ethics and Ethnography in Neonatal Intensive Care," in *Social Science Perspectives*, ed. Weisz, 261–72.

30. Zaner's *Ethics and the Clinical Encounter* is a partial exception, as is Edwin M. Hartman's *Organizational Ethics and the Good Life* (New York: Oxford University Press, 1996). Hartman, significantly, has a joint appointment in the departments of Management and Philosophy at Rutgers.

31. In explaining why medical anthropologists have paid limited attention to medical ethics, Lieban suggests part of it is due to the fact that "cultural relativism has in some form been characteristic of anthropology. This has meant studying other cultures on their own terms and avoiding ethnocentric value judgments about them," Lieban, "Medical Anthropology," in *Social Science Perspectives*, ed. Weisz, 221.

32. Hoffmaster, "Can Ethnography," and Jennings, "Ethics and Ethnography."

33. See *Sociological Methods and Research* (Special Issue on the Value-Added Contributions of Ethnographic Research) 25, no. 4 (May 1997).

34. Susan E. Kelly et al., "Understanding the Practice of Ethics Consultation: Results of an Ethnographic Multi-Site Study," *Journal of Clinical Ethics* 8, no. 2 (Summer 1997): 137. Kelly et al. borrow this definition from Clifford Geertz, *The Interpretation of Cultures* (New York: Basic Books, 1973). In a later work Geertz calls into question the possibility of an outsider being able truly to see the world "from the

native's point of view," at least while also maintaining one's prior critical perspective. See his *Local Knowledge: Further Essays in Interpretive Anthropology* (New York: Basic Books, 1983), especially 55–58.

35. Crigger, "Bioethnography," provides the best starting point for such sources. To her list I would add Bosk, *Forgive and Remember*; Katz Rothman, *In Labor: Women and Power in the Birthplace* (New York: W. W. Norton, 1982); and Sue Fisher and Alexandra Dundas Todd, eds., *The Social Organization of Doctor-Patient Communication*, 2nd ed. (Greenwich, CT: Ablex Publishing, 1993). Journal articles include Celine Marsden, "Care Giver Fidelity in a Pediatric Bone Marrow Transplant Team," *Heart & Lung* 17, no. 6, pt. 1 (November 1988): 617–25; Kelly, "Understanding the Practice"; Jennings, "Ethics and Ethnography"; and Robertson, "Ethical Theory."

36. Gillon, "Ethnography, Medical Practice," 259–60.

37. Michael Polanyi sums it up as, "I shall reconsider human knowledge by starting from the fact that we can know more than we can tell." *The Tacit Dimension* (Garden City, NY: Doubeday & Company, 1966), 4.

38. Zaner, *Clinical Encounter*, 9.

39. Robert Veatch's contract-based *A Theory of Medical Ethics* (New York: Basic Books, 1981) is emblematic of this approach.

40. Hoffmaster, "Can Ethnography," 1425, and see Schneider, *The Practice of Autonomy*.

41. Charmaz and Olesen, "Ethnographic Research," 476–77.

42. Three recent, if very different, scandals reinforce this point—the Los Angeles Police Department Rampart Division, the collapse at Enron, and the abuse of prisoners at Abu Ghraib.

43. Jennings, "Ethics and Ethnography," 269.

44. Jennings, "Ethics and Ethnography," 269. Stackhouse reaches a similarly strong conclusion: "One of the distinctive tasks of ethics is to define the ethos; that is, to identify, to evaluate, to arrange or rearrange those networks of norms that obtain in a sociocultural setting," *Ethics and the Urban Ethos*, 5, emphasis added.

45. Werhane, *Moral Imagination*, 67.

46. On most accounts of moral theory and of the role of the ethicist, the different scheme would include a detailed understanding of universal—not schematized—moral principles. I leave aside whether this is necessary or possible, since, in either case, the ethicist should at least be able to point to a *different* scheme, one, at the minimum, with broader social sanction.

47. Meyers, "Ethics Consulting."

48. See Werhane, "The Normative/Descriptive Distinction in Methodologies of Business Ethics," *Business Ethics Quarterly* 4, no. 2 (April 1994): 175–80.

# Index

~

# About the Author

**Christopher Meyers** is professor of philosophy and director of the Kegley Institute of Ethics at CSU Bakersfield. He is also a member of the medical staff at Kern Medical Center, where he provides ethics consulting and education, services he also provides for most of the major hospitals in the Bakersfield area. Most of his research is in practical ethics, particularly bioethics and journalism ethics.